*Stedman's*

# CARDIOLOGY
# WORDS

STEDMANS

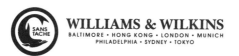

**WILLIAMS & WILKINS**
BALTIMORE · HONG KONG · LONDON · MUNICH
PHILADELPHIA · SYDNEY · TOKYO

*Series Editor:* Elizabeth Randolph
*Editor:* Betsy Dearborn
*Production Manager:* Cordelia Slaughter
*Cover Design:* Carla Frank

Copyright © 1993
Williams & Wilkins
428 East Preston Street
Baltimore, Maryland 21202, USA

*Printed in the United States of America*


**Library of Congress Cataloging-in-Publication Data**
Stedman's cardiology words.
    p.  cm.
  Developed from the database of Stedman's medical dictionary 25th ed. and supplemented by terminology found in the current medical literature.
  Includes bibliographical references.
  ISBN 0-683-07953-0
  1. Cardiology—Terminology.  2. Heart—Diseases—Terminology.
I. Stedman, Thomas Lathrop, 1853–1983. Medical dictionary.
II. Title: Cardiology words.
  [DNLM: 1. Cardiology—terminology.  WG 15 S812]
RC666.3.S74  1992
616.1′2′0014—dc20
DNLM/DLC
for Library of Congress                      92-21067
                                      CIP


92  93  94  95  96
3  4  5  6  7  8  9  10

# *Contents*

# *Acknowledgments*

An important part of our editorial process is the involvement of medical transcriptionists—as advisors, reviewers, and/or editors. Betsy Dearborn of Arlington, Virginia, did an excellent job of editing and proofing the manuscript, and didn't miss a deadline! Harriet Stewart, CMT, and Donna Taylor, CMT, also contributed their word research and editorial expertise to the project.

Special thanks go to the members of the Williams & Wilkins MT Advisory Board, whose expertise, ideas, and words contribute to the overall quality of this and other *Stedman's* word books: LaVonne Alexis, CMT; Joan Bachman; Addie M. Garner; Suzanne Minnick, CMT; Susan Pierce, CMT, ART; Laurie J. Spangler, CMT; Harriet Stewart, CMT; and Dorothy Vickers.

# Explanatory Notes

*Stedman's Cardiology Words* offers an authoritative assurance of quality and exactness to the wordsmiths of the health care professions—medical transcriptionists, medical editors and copy editors, medical records personnel, and the many other users and producers of medical documentation. It can be used to validate both the spelling and accuracy of terminology in cardiology. This compilation of over 18,000 entries, fully cross-indexed for quick access, was built from a base vocabulary of medical words, phrases, abbreviations, and acronyms. The extensive A–Z list was developed from the database of *Stedman's Medical Dictionary, 25ed.* and supplemented by terminology found in the current medical literature.

Medical transcription is an art as well as a science. Both are needed to correctly interpret a physician's dictation, whose language is a product of education, training, and experience. This variety in medical language means that there are several acceptable ways to express certain terms, including jargon. *Stedman's Cardiology Words* provides variant spellings and phrasings for many terms. This, in addition to complete cross-indexing, makes *Stedman's Cardiology Words* a valuable resource for determining the validity of cardiology terms as they are encountered.

*Stedman's Cardiology Words* includes up-to-date terminology of medical and surgical therapy, diagnostic modalities and imaging techniques, cardiac catheterization, angiography, electrophysiology of the heart, rehabilitation, and exercise. The user will find listed thousands of diseases and syndromes, abbreviations, eponyms, and diagnostic tests and procedures. Equipment and drug names related to the specialty are also included. An appendix at the back of the book matches select cardiology procedures with related medical terminology.

## Alphabetical Organization

Alphabetization of entries is letter by letter as spelled, ignoring punctuation, spaces, prefixed numbers, Greek letters, or other characters. For example:

**acid-fast staining methods**
**acid formaldehyde hematin**
**$\alpha_1$-acid glycoprotein**
**acid hematin**

In subentries, the abbreviated singular form or the spelled-out plural form of the noun main entry word is ignored in alphabetization.

## Format and Style

All main entries are in **boldface** to speed up location of a sought-after entry, to enhance distinction between main entries and subentries, and to relieve the textual density of the pages.

Irregular plurals and variant spellings are shown on the same line as the singular or preferred form of the word. For example:

**myxoma, pl. myxomata**

**ectasia, ectasis**
    annuloaortic e.
    artery e.
    e. cordis

Possessive forms that occur in the medical literature are retained in this reference. It should be noted that eponymic equipment and instrument names frequently appear in non-possessive form. To form the non-possessives advocated by the American Association for Medical Transcription and other groups, simply drop the apostrophe or apostrophe "s" from the end of the word.

## Cross-indexing

The word list is in an index-like main entry-subentry format that contains two combined alphabetical listings:

(1) a noun main entry-subentry organization typical of the A-Z section of medical dictionaries like *Stedman's*:

**ablation**
catheter a.
continuous wave laser a.
electrical a.
laser a.

**edema**
alveolar e.
angioneurotic e.
cardiac e.
cardiogenic pulmonary e.

(2) An adjective main entry-subentry organization, which lists words and phrases as you hear them. The main entries are the adjectives or descriptors in a multi-word term. The subentries are the nouns around which the terms are constructed and to which the adjectives or descriptors pertain:

**cardiac**
c. accident
c. amyloidosis
c. aneurysm
c. apex

**mesenteric**
m. angiography
m. arteritis
m. artery occlusion
m. bypass graft

This format provides the user with more than one way to locate and identify a multi-word term. For example:

**needle**
Brockenbrough n.

**Brockenbrough**
B. needle

**tachycardia**
ectopic atrial t.

**ectopic**
e. atrial tachycardia

It also allows the user to see together all terms that contain a particular modifier as well as all types, kinds, or variations of a noun entity. For example:

**aneurysm**
abdominal aortic a.
a. by anastomosis
aortic a.
arteriovenous a.

**circulatory**
c. arrest
c. collapse
c. congestion
c. failure

**catheter**
c. ablation
ACS angioplasty c.
ACS balloon c.
AL II guiding c.

Abbreviations are defined and cross-referenced throughout. For example:

**ECLA**
excimer laser coronary angioplasty

**angioplasty**
excimer laser coronary a. (ECLA)

**excimer**
e. laser coronary angioplasty (ECLA)

## References

Bashore, Percutaneous balloon valvuloplasty and related techniques. Baltimore: Williams & Wilkins, 1991.

Braundwald, Cardiovascular disease, 4th ed. Philadelphia: W.B. Saunders, 1992.

Catheterization and cardiovascular diagnosis. New York: Wiley-Liss, 1991.

FDA. Medical device registration master file. Rockville, MD: Food and Drug Administration, 1991.

Feigenbaum, Echocardiography, 4th ed. Malvern, PA: Lea & Febiger, 1986.

Grossman, Cardiac catheterization, angiography and intervention. Malvern, PA: Lea & Febiger, 1991.

Hurst, The heart, 7th ed. New York: McGraw-Hill, 1990.

Journal of interventional cardiology. Mount Kisco, NY: Futura, 1990.

Lubell, The cath lab. Baltimore: Williams & Wilkins, 1990.

Marriott, Practical electrocardiography, 8th ed. Baltimore: Williams & Wilkins, 1988.

Opie, Drugs for the heart, 2nd ed. Philadelphia: W.B. Saunders, 1987.

Pepine, Diagnostic and therapeutic cardiac catheterization. Baltimore: Williams & Wilkins, 1989.

Stedman's abbreviations, acronyms and symbols. Baltimore: Williams & Wilkins, 1992.

Stedman's medical dictionary, 25th ed. Baltimore: Williams & Wilkins, 1990.

## Your Medical Word Resource Publisher

We strive to provide you with the most up-to-date and accurate word references available. Your use of this word book will prompt new editions, which will be published as often as justified by updates and revisions. We welcome your suggestions for improvements, changes, corrections, and additions—whatever will make this **Stedman's** product more useful to you. Please use the postpaid card at the back of this book and send your recommendations to the Reference Division at Williams & Wilkins.

α$_2$-plasmin inhibitor
**AA**
 ascending aorta
**AAA**
 abdominal aortic aneurysm
**AAI pacing**
**AAIR pacing**
**AAI-RR pacing**
**AAT pacing**
**abacterial thrombotic endocarditis**
**Abbott infusion pump**
**ABC leads**
**abdominal**
 a. angina
 a. aorta
 a. aortic aneurysm (AAA)
 a. aortography
 a. bruit
**abdominocardiac reflex**
**abdominojugular reflux**
**abdominothoracic pump**
**aberrancy**
 acceleration-dependent a.
 bradycardia-dependent a.
 postextrasystolic a.
 tachycardia-dependent a.
**aberrant**
 a. artery
 a. complex
 a. conduction
 a. ventricular conduction
**aberration**
 intraventricular a.
 ventricular a.
**abetalipoproteinemia**
 familial a.
**ablation**
 catheter a.
 continuous-wave laser a.
 electrical a.

 laser a.
 pulsed laser a.
 surgical a.
 tissue a.
**ablative**
 a. cardiac surgery
 a. laser angioplasty
 a. technique
**abnormal**
 a. cleavage of cardiac valve
 a. left axis deviation (ALAD)
 a. right axis deviation (ARAD)
**abnormality**
 atrioventricular conduction a.
 clotting a.
 electrical activation a.
 figure-of-eight a.
 hemodynamic a.
 left ventricular wall motion a.
 sinus node/AV conduction a.
 ventricular depolarization a.
**aborted systole**
**abouchement**
**Abrams' heart reflex**
**abscess**
 aortic root a.
 brain a.
 embolic a.
 myocardial a.
 papillary muscle a.
 periaortic a.
**absent pericardium**
**absolute refractory period**
**abuse**
 alcohol a.

**abuse** *(continued)*
    cocaine a.
    drug a.
**acanthocytosis**
**acapnia**
**acarbia**
**acardiotrophia**
**ACC**
    American College of
    Cardiology
**accelerated**
    a. conduction
    a. idioventricular rhythm
    a. junctional rhythm
**accelerated-malignant**
  **hypertension**
**acceleration-dependent**
  **aberrancy**
**acceleration time**
**access**
    venous a.
**accessory**
    a. artery
    a. atrium
    a. pathway
**accident**
    cardiac a.
    cardiovascular a.
    cerebrovascular a. (CVA)
**accidental murmur**
**accretio cordis**
**accrochage**
**Accufix pacemaker**
**Acculith pacemaker**
**accumulation**
    phytanic acid a.
**Accupril**
**Accuretic**
**ACE**
    angiotensin-converting
    enzyme
      ACE inhibitor
**acebutolol**
**acebutolol HCl**

**acecainide**
**acetate**
    desmopressin a.
    (DDAVP)
**acetazolamide**
**acetylcarnitine**
**acetylcholine test**
**acetyl CoA**
**acetyldigitoxin**
***N*-acetylprocainamide**
**acetylsalicylic acid**
**ACG**
    apex impulse tracing
**acid**
    acetylsalicylic a.
    amino a.
    aminocaproic a.
    aminosalicylic a.
    arachidonic a.
    ascorbic a.
    chenodeoxycholic a.
    deoxyribonucleic a.
    (DNA)
    digammacarboxy-
     glutamic a.
    docosahexaenoic a.
    eicosapentaenoic a.
    ethacrynic a.
    fatty a.
    fibric a.
    folic a.
    glycyrrhizinic a.
    hydrocyanic a.
    a. infusion test
    lactic a.
    linoleic a.
    a. maltase deficiency
    a. mucopolysaccharide
    (AMP)
    nicotinic a.
    omega-3 unsaturated
     fatty a.
    palmitic a.

para-aminosalicylic a.
  (PAS, PASA)
pyruvic a.
ribonucleic a. (RNA)
uric a.
**acid-base imbalance**
**acidemia**
**acidity**
  total a.
**acidosis**
  hyperchloremic a.
  metabolic a.
*Acinetobacter calcoaceticus*
**a-c interval**
**acleistocardia**
**acoustic**
  a. imaging
  a. impedance
  a. shadow
**acquired immunodeficiency**
  **syndrome (AIDS)**
**acquisition**
  multiple gated a.
  (MUGA)
**acrocyanosis**
**acromegaly**
**acrotic**
**acrotism**
**ACS**
  Alcon Closure System
  American Cancer Society
  American College of
  Surgeons
  ACS Angioject
  ACS angioplasty catheter
  ACS angioplasty Y-
  connector
  ACS balloon catheter
  ACS LIMA guide
  ACS microglide wire
  ACS percutaneous
  introducer set
  ACS RX coronary
  dilatation catheter

**ACTH**
  adrenocorticotropic
  hormone
**α-actin**
**α-actinin**
*Actinobacillus*
  *actinomycetemcomitans*
*Actinomyces israelii*
*actinomycetemcomitans*
  *Actinobacillus a.*
**actinomycosis**
**action**
  catecholamine a.
  mechanism of a.
  a. potential
**Activase**
**activated partial**
  **thromboplastin time (APTT,**
  **AtPP)**
**activation**
  length-dependent a.
**activator**
  plasminogen a.
  recombinant tissue
  plasminogen a. (rt-PA)
  tissue plasminogen a.
  (tPA, t-PA)
**active**
  a. congestion
  a. dynamic stiffness
  a. hyperemia
**Activitrax pacemaker**
**activity**
  intrinsic
  sympathomimetic a.
  (ISA)
  membrane-stabilizing a.
  physical a.
  a. scale
  sexual a.
  triggered a.
**activity-sensing pacemaker**
**actuarial survival curve**

3

**acuity**
> visual a.

**acute**
> a. bacterial endocarditis
> a. compression triad
> a. glomerulonephritis
> (AGN)
> a. intermittent porphyria
> a. isolated myocarditis
> a. myocardial infarction
> (AMI)
> a. pericarditis
> a. renal failure
> a. respiratory failure
> (ARF)
> a. response
> a. rheumatic arthritis
> a. rheumatic fever
> (ARF)
> a. tamponade

**acyanotic**
**acylcarnitine**
**acyl cholesterol acyltransferase**
**inhibitor**
**acyl CoA**
**acyl-coenzyme A**
**acyltransferase**
> lecithin-cholesterol a.
> (LCAT)

**Adalat**
**Adams-DeWeese device**
**Adams-Stokes**
> A.-S. disease
> A.-S. syncope
> A.-S. syndrome

**adapter**
> catheter a.
> Harris a.
> Tuohy-Bost a.

**Addison's**
> A. disease
> A. maneuver

**Adenocard**

**Adenoscan**
**adenosine**
> a. deaminase
> a. diphosphate (ADP)
> a. monophosphate
> (AMP)
> a. thallium test
> a. triphosphate (ATP)

**adenosinetriphosphatase**
**(ATPase)**
**adenovirus**
**adenylate**
> a. cyclase
> a. cyclase system

**ADH**
> antidiuretic hormone

**adherent pericardium**
**adhesive pericarditis**
**adiastole**
**adiemorrhysis**
**adipose tissue**
**adiposis**
> a. cardiaca
> a. universalis

**admixture**
**ADP**
> adenosine diphosphate

**adrenal**
> a. gland
> a. hyperplasia
> a. hypertension
> a. medulla
> a. vein aldosterone

**adrenaline**
**adrenergic**
> α-a., alpha-a.
> a. adrenergic
> β-a. stimulation
> a. antagonist
> β-a., beta-a.
> a. nervous system
> a. receptor
> a. stimulant

adrenoceptor blocker
adrenocorticotropic hormone
  (ACTH)
adrenogenital syndrome
adrenoreceptor
Adriamycin cardiotoxicity
Adson forceps
adultorum
    scleredema a.
adult respiratory distress
  syndrome (ARDS)
advanced life support (ALS)
adventitia
AE-60-I-2 implantable pronged
  unipolar electrode
AE-60-K-10 implantable
  unipolar endocardial
  electrode
AE-60-KB implantable
  unipolar endocardial
  electrode
AE-60-KS-10 implantable
  unipolar endocardial
  electrode
AE-85-I-2 implantable pronged
  unipolar electrode
AE-85-K-10 implantable
  unipolar endocardial
  electrode
AE-85-KB implantable
  unipolar endocardial
  electrode
AE-85-KS-10 implantable
  unipolar endocardial
  electrode
aeremia
aerendocardia
aerobic
    a. capacity
    a. metabolism
*Aerococcus viridans*
*aeruginosa*
    *Pseudomonas a.*
AES Amplatz guide wire

afferent impulse
affinity
afflux, affluxion
AFORMED
    alternating, failure of
    response, mechanical, to
    electrical depolarization
    AFORMED phenomenon
African
    A. cardiomyopathy
    A. sleeping sickness
afterdepolarization
    delayed a.
    early a.
afterload
    a. matching
    a. mismatching
    a. reduction
    a. resistance
    ventricular a.
afterpotential
    diastolic a.
    oscillatory a.
Ag
    silver
age
    chronologic a. (CA)
agent
    alpha blocking a.
    antianginal a.
    antiarrhythmic a.
    antidiabetic a.
    antihypertensive a.
    antiplatelet a.
    antipsychotic a.
    beta blocking a.
    calcium channel
      blocking a.
    contraceptive a.
    contrast a.
    dopaminergic a.
    hypoglycemic a.
    inhalation a.
    inotropic a.

5

*Alfieri repair*

**agent** *(continued)*
    nonglycoside inotropic a.
    nonsteroidal
      antiinflammatory a.
    psychotropic a.
    thrombolytic a.
    toxic a.
    vasodilator a.
**agglutinating antibody**
**agglutinative thrombus**
**aglycone**
**AGN**
    acute glomerulonephritis
**agonal**
    a. rhythm
    a. thrombus
**agonist**
    alpha a.
    alpha-adrenoreceptor a.
    beta a.
    beta-adrenoreceptor a.
    calcium channel a.
**agony clot**
**agranulocytosis**
**A-H**
    A-H conduction time
    A-H interval
**AHA**
    American Heart Association
**AICD**
    automatic implantable
    cardioverter-defibrillator
**AIDS**
    acquired immunodeficiency
    syndrome
**air**
    a. clamp inflatable
      vessel occluder
    a. embolism
    a. embolization
    a. embolus
    a. pulmonary embolism
    a. saw
**air-driven artificial heart**

**airway clearance**
**akinesia**
**akinesis**
**akinetic**
**Al**
    aluminum
**ALAD**
    abnormal left axis deviation
**alanine**
**alanine aminotransferase**
  **(ALT)**
**Albini's nodule**
**Albright's syndrome**
**albumin**
**albuterol**
**alcohol**
    a. abuse
    ethyl a.
    a. intoxication
**alcoholic**
    a. cardiomyopathy
    a. malnutrition
**Alcon Closure System (ACS)**
**Aldactazide**
**Aldactone**
**Aldomet**
**aldosterone**
    adrenal vein a.
    a. antagonist
    a. depression
**aldosteronism**
**aldosteronoma**
**alfentanil**
**algiovascular**
**algorithm**
**algovascular**
**aliasing**
**alignment mark**
**AL II guiding catheter**
**alkaloid**
    ergot a.
    *Rauwolfia* a.
**alkalosis**
    metabolic a.

**alkaptonuria**
**allantoic vein**
**allele**
    mutant a.
**Allen test**
**allergic granulomatosis**
**allergy**
**Allis clamp**
**all or none**
**allogeneic transplantation**
**allograft**
**allorhythmia**
**allorhythmic**
**allosteric modification of**
  **enzyme**
**alpha**
    a. agonist
    a. blocking agent
    a. lipoprotein
    a. receptor
**alpha-adrenergic blocker**
**alpha-adrenoreceptor**
    a.-a. agonist
    a.-a. blocker
**alpha-methyldopa**
**Alport's syndrome**
**alprazolam**
**alprenolol**
**ALS**
    advanced life support
**ALT**
    alanine aminotransferase
**Altace**
**alternans**
    auditory a.
    auscultatory a.
    concordant a.
    discordant a.
    electrical a.
    parvus a.
    pulsus a.
    QRS a.
    ST segment a.

    total a.
    U wave a.
**alternating, failure of**
  **response, mechanical, to**
  **electrical depolarization**
  **(AFORMED)**
**alternating pulse**
**alternation**
    concordant a.
    discordant a.
    electrical a. of heart
    a. of heart
    mechanical a.
**alterplase recombinant**
**altitude**
    high a.
    a. hypoxia
**aluminum (Al)**
**aluminum hydroxide gel**
**alveolar**
    a. edema
    a. hypoventilation
    a. hypoxia
    a. proteinosis
    a. tension
**alveolar-capillary membrane**
**alveolocapillary membrane**
**amaurosis fugax**
**ambiguus**
    situs a.
**ambulation**
**ambulatory**
    a. electrocardiography
    a. monitoring
**amebiasis**
**ameboid cell**
**American**
    A. Cancer Society
    (ACS)
    A. College of
    Cardiology (ACC)
    A. College of Surgeons
    (ACS)

**American** *(continued)*
    A. Heart Association (AHA)
    A. Heart Association diet
**AMI**
    acute myocardial infarction
**Amidate**
**amiloride**
**amine**
    sympathomimetic a.
**amino acid**
**aminocaproic acid**
**aminoglycoside**
**aminophylline**
**aminorex**
**aminosalicylic**
    a. acid
    a. acid hypersensitivity
**aminotransferase**
    alanine a. (ALT)
    aspartate a. (AST)
**amiodarone**
**amiodarone-induced hyperthyroidism**
**Amipaque**
**amitriptyline**
**amlodipine**
**ammonia**
    N-13 a.
    nitrogen-13 a.
**ammonium chloride**
**amniocentesis**
**amniotic**
    a. fluid embolism
    a. fluid pulmonary embolism
    a. fluid syndrome
**A-mode echocardiography**
**amoxapine**
**amoxicillin**
**AMP**
    acid mucopolysaccharide

    average mean pressure
    adenosine monophosphate
**ampere**
**amphetamine**
    a. toxicity
**amphipathic helix**
**Amphojel**
**amphotericin B**
**ampicillin**
**Amplatz**
    A. catheter
    A. coronary catheter
    A. high-flo torque control catheter
    A. technique
**Amplex guide wire**
**amplitude**
    apical interventricular septal a.
    atrial pulse a.
    C to E a.
    D to E a.
    a. image
    a. linearity
    a. of pulse
    P-wave a.
    R-wave a.
    ventricular pulse a.
    wall a.
**ampulla**, gen. and pl. **ampullae**
    Bryant's a.
    Thoma's a.
**amrinone**
    a. lactate
**amsacrine**
**amylase**
**amyl nitrite**
**amyloid heart disease**
**amyloidosis**
    cardiac a.
    familial a.
    senile a.
**amyocardia**
**amyotrophic chorea**

**ANA**
    antinuclear antibody
**anabolic steroid**
**anacrotic**
    a. limb
    a. limb pulse
    a. notch
    a. pulse
**anacrotism**
**anadicrotic pulse**
**anadicrotism**
**anaerobic**
    a. metabolism
    a. threshold
**analgesia**
**analgesic nephropathy**
**analog-to-digital conversion**
**analysis**
    centerline method of
      wall motion a.
    cost-benefit a.
    cost-effectiveness a.
    Fourier a.
    Fourier series a.
    Fourier transform a.
    pressure-volume a.
    probability a.
    sensitivity a.
    wall motion a.
**analyzer**
    Criticare ETCO2
      multigas a.
    Datex ETCO2
      multigas a.
    ETCO2 multigas a.
    Nellcor N2500 ETCO2
      multigas a.
    Novametrix ETCO2
      multigas a.
    Ohmeda ETCO2
      multigas a.
    pacing system a.
    pulse-height a.

    Puritan Bennett ETCO2
      multigas a.
**anangioplasia**
**anangioplastic**
**anapamil**
**anaphylactoid**
    a. purpura
    a. reaction
**anaphylatoxin**
**anaphylaxis**
**anastomosis, pl. anastomoses**
    aneurysm by a.
    arteriovenous a.
    portacaval a.
    Potts' a.
    systemic-to-pulmonary
      artery a.
**anatomic**
    a. assessment
    a. localization
**anatricrotic**
**anatricrotism**
**ANCOR imaging system**
**Ancrod**
**Anectine**
    A. chloride
**anemia**
    aplastic a.
    chronic hemolytic a.
    Cooley's a.
    hemolytic a.
    Mediterranean a.
    megaloblastic a.
    microangiopathic a.
    sickle cell a.
    splenic a.
**anemic murmur**
**anesthesia**
    Bier block a.
    epidural a.
    general a.
    local a.
    regional a.
    spinal a.

**anesthesiology**
**anesthetic**
**aneurysm**
abdominal aortic a.
(AAA)
a. by anastomosis
aortic a.
arteriovenous a.
atherosclerotic a.
atrial septal a.
brain a.
cardiac a.
cirsoid a.
coronary a.
Crisp's a.
dissecting aortic a.
embolic a.
embolomycotic a.
false a.
false aortic a.
fusiform a.
infected a.
infrarenal abdominal
aortic a.
interventricular
septum a.
left ventricular a.
mitral valve a.
mural a.
mycotic a.
mycotic aortic a.
phantom a.
Pott's a.
racemose a.
saccular a.
Shekelton's a.
sinus of Valsalva a.
syphilitic a.
thoracoabdominal
aortic a.
traction a.
traumatic a.
traumatic aortic a.

true aortic a.
ventricular a.
**aneurysmal, aneurysmatic**
a. bruit
a. hematoma
a. phthisis
**aneurysmectomy**
**ANF**
atrial natriuretic factor
**Anger**
A. camera
A. scintillation camera
**Angestat hemostasis introducer**
**Angetear tearaway introducer**
**angialgia**
**angiasthenia**
**angiitis**
leukocytoelastic a.
necrotizing a.
**angina**
abdominal a.
Canadian Cardiovascular
Society grading of a.
chronic a.
chronic stable a.
a. cordis
crescendo a.
a. decubitus
a. of effort
effort a.
exertional a.
false a.
Heberden's a.
hypercyanotic a.
a. inversa
nonexertional a.
a. notha
a. pectoris
a. pectoris decubitus
a. pectoris sine dolore
a. pectoris vasomotoria
postinfarction a.
Prinzmetal's a.
reflex a.

rest a.
a. sine dolore
a. spuria
stable a.
unstable a.
variant a.
variant a. pectoris
vasomotor a., a.
  vasomotoria
walk-through a.
**anginal equivalent**
**anginiform**
**anginoid**
**anginose, anginous**
**angiocardiogram**
**angiocardiography**
first-pass radionuclide a.
radionuclide a.
transseptal a.
**angiocardiokinetic**
**angiocardiopathy**
**angiocarditis**
**Angiocath catheter**
**angiodynia**
**angiodysplasia**
a. of colon
**angioedema**
**Angioflow high-flow catheter**
**angiographic**
a. assessment
a. catheter
a. instrumentation
**angiography**
aortography a.
balloon-occlusion
  pulmonary a.
carotid a.
cerebral a.
coronary a.
digital a.
digital subtraction a.
  (DSA)
fluorescein a.

internal mammary artery
  graft a.
left aortic a.
left atrial a.
left ventricular a.
mesenteric a.
noncardiac a.
nonselective coronary a.
pulmonary a.
pulmonary wedge a.
radionuclide a.
renal a.
renovascular a.
saphenous vein bypass
  graft a.
selective a.
ventricular a.
wedged pulmonary a.
**Angioject**
ACS A.
**angiokeratoma**
a. corporis diffusum
**angiokinesis**
**angioma**
**angionecrosis**
**angioneurotic edema**
**angioplasty**
ablative laser a.
balloon a.
balloon coarctation a.
balloon laser a.
bootstrap two-vessel a.
complex a.
coronary a.
excimer laser
  coronary a. (ECLA,
  ELCA)
a. guiding catheter
high-risk a.
laser a.
percutaneous balloon a.
percutaneous
  transluminal a.

**angioplasty** *(continued)*
    percutaneous
      transluminal
      coronary a. (PTCA)
    peripheral a.
    rescue a.
    routine a.
    thrombolysis and a. in
      myocardial infarction
      (TAMI)
    transluminal a.
    transluminal coronary a.
**angioplasty-related vessel**
  **occlusion**
**angiosarcoma**
**angioscope**
    Masy a.
**angioscopy**
**angiostomy**
**angiotensin**
**angiotensinase**
**angiotensin-converting enzyme**
  **(ACE inhibitor, ACE)**
**angiotomy**
**Angiovist**
**angle**
    costovertebral a. (CVA)
    intercept a.
    Louis' a.
**angled pigtail catheter**
**angor**
    a. animi
    a. pectoris
**Ang-O-Span**
**angulated multipurpose**
  **catheter**
**angulation**
    RAO a.
**Anhydron**
**A-N interval**
**anion exchange resin**
**anisopiesis**
**anisorrhythmia**

**anisosphygmia**
**anisotropy**
**ankle**
    a. blood pressure
    a. exercise
**ankle/brachial index**
**ankylosing spondylitis (AS)**
**annihilation photon**
**annular array transducer**
**annuli**
**annuloaortic ectasia**
**annuloplasty**
    DeVega a.
**annulus, anulus, pl. annuli**
    aortic a.
    a. fibrosi cordis
    a. fibrosis
    mitral a.
    mitral valve a.
    a. ovalis
    tricuspid valve a.
**anodal**
    a. closure contraction
    a. opening contraction
**anomalous**
    a. complex
    a. mitral arcade
    a. origin
    a. pulmonary vein
    a. pulmonary venous
      connection
    a. pulmonary venous
      drainage
    a. pulmonary venous
      return
    a. rectification
**anomaly**
    atrioventricular
      connection a.
    coronary artery a.
    Ebstein's a.
    pulmonary valve a.

pulmonary venous
connection a.
pulmonary venous
return a.
Shone's a.
Taussig-Bing a.
Uhl's a.
ventricular inflow a.
**anorexia nervosa**
**anotia**
**anoxemia test**
**anoxia**
myocardial a.
stagnant a.
**AN region**
**Anrep effect**
**ansa cervicalis**
**antacid**
**antagonist**
adrenergic a.
aldosterone a.
calcium a.
calcium channel a.'s
thromboxane receptor a.
vitamin K a.
**antecubital fossa**
**antegrade**
a. approach
a. conduction
**antegrade/retrograde**
**cardioplegia technique**
**antemortem**
a. clot
a. thrombus
**anterior**
a. approach
a. leaflet
a. myocardial infarction
a. oblique projection
**anterograde**
a. block
a. conduction
**anteroinferior myocardial**
**infarction**

**anterolateral myocardial**
**infarction**
**anteroposterior**
a. projection
a. thoracic diameter
**anteroseptal myocardial**
**infarction**
**antesystole**
**anthracycline**
a. drug
a. toxicity
**anthraquinone**
**antianginal agent**
**antiarrhythmic**
a. agent
a. therapy
**antibiotic**
prophylactic a.
**antibody, pl. antibodies**
agglutinating a.
antinuclear a. (ANA)
B-cell a.
cross-reactive a.
digitalis-specific a.
fibrin-specific a.
monoclonal a.
myosin-specific a.
OKT3 a.
platelet a.
streptococcal a.
streptokinase a.
thyroid a.
treponemal a.
**antibradycardia**
**anticoagulant**
lupus a.
a. therapy
**anticoagulation**
**anti-deoxyribonuclease B**
**antidepressant**
tricyclic a.
**antidiabetic agent**
**antidiuretic hormone (ADH)**
**antidromic tachycardia**

**antidysrhythmic**
**antiembolism stockings**
**antigen**
    human lymphocyte a.
    (HLA)
**antiheart antibody titer**
**antihistamine**
**antihypertensive agent**
**antilymphocyte globulin**
**antimicrobial**
**antimony**
    a. compound
    a. toxicity
**antimyosin infarct-avid**
  **scintigraphy**
**antinuclear antibody (ANA)**
**antiplasmin**
**antiplatelet**
    a. agent
    a. therapy
**antipsychotic agent**
**antishock garment**
**antistreptolysin O (ASO)**
**antistreptozyme (ASTZ)**
**antitachycardia pacemaker**
  **(ATP)**
**antithrombin**
**antithrombin III (AT-III)**
**antithrombotic**
**antithymocyte**
    a. globulin
**antituberculous drug**
**Anturane**
**anulus** (*var. of* annulus)
**anxiety**
    a. attack
    a. neurosis
**AOO pacing**
**aorta**, gen. and pl. **aortae**
    abdominal a.
    a. angusta
    ascending a. (AA)
    bifurcation of a.
    buckled a.

    coarctation of a.
    descending a.
    dissection of a.
    dynamic a.
    kinked a.
    overriding a.
    recoarctation of a.
    thoracic a.
**aorta-femoral artery shunt**
**aorta-left atrium ratio**
**aortalgia**
**aortarctia**
**aortartia**
**aortectasis, aortectasia**
**aortectomy**
**aortic**
    a. aneurysm
    a. aneurysmal disease
    a. aneurysm clamp
    a. annulus
    a. arch
    a. arch interruption
    a. arch syndrome
    a. arteritis syndrome
    a. atresia
    a. clamp
    a. coarctation
    a. crossclamp
    a. cusp separation
    a. dissection
    a. dwarfism
    a. embolism
    a. facies
    a. homograft
    a. impedance
    a. incompetence
    a. insufficiency
    a. jet velocity
    a. knob
    a. murmur
    a. notch
    a. obstruction
    a. perfusion cannula
    a. pressure

a. pressure gradient
a. prosthesis
a. pullback pressure
a. reflex
a. regurgitation
a. regurgitation murmur
a. restenosis
a. root
a. root abscess
a. rupture
a. sac
a. sclerosis
a. septal defect
a. sinus
a. spindle
a. stenosis (AS)
a. stenosis murmur
a. thromboembolic
 disease
a. thrombosis
a. valve
a. valve area
a. valve disease
a. valve gradient
a. valve leaflet
a. valve replacement
 (AVR)
a. valve resistance
a. valve restenosis
a. valve vegetation
a. valve velocity profile
a. valvotomy
a. valvular insufficiency
a. valvulitis
a. valvuloplasty
a. valvulotomy
a. window
**aortic aneurysm**
 abdominal a.a. (AAA)
 congenital a.a.
 dissecting a.a.
 false a.a.
 fusiform a.a.
 infrarenal abdominal a.a.

mycotic a.a.
ruptured a.a.
saccular a.a.
syphilitic a.a.
thoracic a.a.
thoracoabdominal a.a.
traumatic a.a.
**aortic arch**
 cervical a. a.
 circumflex a. a.
 double a. a.
 interrupted a. a.
 a. a. interruption
**aortic cusp separation**
**aortic-left ventricular tunnel**
 **murmur**
**aortic-mitral combined disease**
 **murmur**
**aorticopulmonary**
 a. defect
 a. septal defect
 a. window
**aorticus**
 torus a.
**aortic valve**
 bicuspid a.v.
 St. Jude prosthetic a.v.
**aortismus abdominalis**
**aortitis**
 arthritis-associated a.
 giant cell a.
 luetic a.
 rheumatic a.
 syphilitic a.
**aortobifemoral**
**aortocaval fistula**
**aortocoronary bypass**
**aortofemoral**
 a. bypass
 a. bypass graft
**aortography**
 abdominal a.
 a. angiography
 ascending a.

**aortography** *(continued)*
    atherosclerotic a.
    biplane a.
    Marfan's syndrome a.
    mycotic a.
    single-plane a.
    sinus of Valsalva a.
    translumbar a.
    traumatic a.
    true vs. false
      aneurysm a.
**aortoiliac**
    a. bypass
    a. bypass graft
    a. occlusive disease
    a. thrombosis
**aortopathy**
**aortoplasty**
**aortoptosia, aortoptosis**
**aortopulmonary**
    a. collateral
    a. fenestration
    a. window
**aortorrhaphy**
**aortosclerosis**
**aortostenosis**
**aortotomy**
**apathetic hyperthyroidism**
**APB**
    atrial premature beat
**APC**
    atrial premature complexes
**Apert's syndrome**
**aperture**
    transducer a.
**apex**
    a. beat
    cardiac a.
    a. cardiogram
    a. cardiography
    a. cordis
    a. impulse
    a. impulse testing

    a. impulse tracing
    (ACG)
**apex cardiogram**
    hyperdynamic a. c.
**apical**
    a. examination
    a. interventricular septal
      amplitude
    a. left ventricular
      puncture
    a. mid-diastolic heart
      murmur
    a. systolic heart murmur
    a. view
**aplastic anemia**
**apnea**
    obstructive sleep a.
    (OSA)
    sleep a.
**apolipoprotein**
**apolipoprotein B**
**apolipoprotein D**
**apolipoprotein E**
**apoplexy**
**apoprotein**
**apoprotein E**
**appendage**
    atrial a.
    auricular a.
    left atrial a.
    right atrial a.
**appendectomy**
    auricular a.
**approach**
    antegrade a.
    anterior a.
    brachial a.
    brachial artery a.
    central a.
    femoral a.
    percutaneous a.
    posterior a.
    retrograde a.
    retrograde femoral a.

**approximator**
rib a.
**Apresazide**
**Apresoline**
**Aprinox**
**apron**
lead a.
**aprotinin**
**APTT**
activated partial
thromboplastin time
**Aquatag**
**Aquazide**
**Aquazide H**
**arabinoside**
cytosine a. (CA)
**arachidonic acid**
**arachnodactyly**
**ARAD**
abnormal right axis
deviation
**aramine**
**Arani catheter**
**Arantius' nodule**
**arborization block**
**arbovirus**
**arcade**
anomalous mitral a.
**arch**
aortic a.
congenital interrupted
aortic a.
interrupted aortic a.
palmar a.
right aortic a.
**arcus cornae**
**ARDS**
adult respiratory distress
syndrome
**area**, pl. **areae, areas**
aortic valve a.
body surface a. (BSA)
a. of cardiac dullness

effective balloon
dilating a. (EBDA)
mitral a.
mitral valve a. (MVA)
pulmonary a.
pulmonary valve a.
subxiphoid a.
tricuspid a.
tricuspid valve a.
truncoconal a.
valve a.
valve orifice a.
**area-length method**
**Arelix**
**ARF**
acute respiratory failure
acute rheumatic fever
**Arfonad**
**arginine vasopressin**
**argon**
a. laser
a. needle
a. vessel dilator
**Argyle catheter**
**Argyll Robertson pupils**
**armored heart**
**array**
multi-element linear a.
**arrest**
asystolic a.
bradyarrhythmic a.
cardiac a. (CA)
cardiopulmonary a.
circulatory a.
cold ischemic a.
deep hypothermia
circulatory a. (DHCA)
in-hospital cardiac a.
out-of-hospital cardiac a.
sinus a.
total circulatory a.
**arrhythmia**
atrial a.
cardiac a.

17

**arrhythmia** *(continued)*
    juvenile a.
    lethal a.
    malignant ventricular a.
    nodal a.
    nonphasic sinus a.
    phasic a.
    phasic sinus a.
    respiratory a.
    sinus a.
    supraventricular a.
    ventricular a.
**arrhythmic**
**arrhythmogenesis**
**arrhythmogenic**
    a. right ventricular
      dysplasia
**arrhythmokinesis**
**Arrow**
    A. balloon wedge
      catheter
    A. Berman angiographic
      balloon
    A.-Howes catheter
    A. sheath
    A. Twin Catheter
**arsenic (As)**
    a. poisoning
**arsine gas poisoning**
**arteria**, gen. and pl. **arteriae**
**arterial**
    a. blood flow
    a. blood gases
    a. calcification
    a. coupling
    a. cutdown
    a. dissection
    a. embolectomy catheter
    a. entry site
    a. filter
    a. hyperemia
    a. hypotension
    a. hypoxemia
    a. impedance

    a. insufficiency
    a. line
    a. media
    a. murmur
    a. needle
    a. oscillator
      endarterectomy
      instrument
    a. pressure
    a. pulse
    a. sclerosis
    a. sheath
    a. spasm
    a. switch operation
    a. thrombosis
    a. wave
**arterialization**
**arterial-venous oxygen content**
  **difference**
**arteriarctia**
**arteriectasis, arteriectasia**
**arteries**
**arterioatony**
**arteriocapillary sclerosis**
**arteriographic**
**arteriography**
    catheter a.
    coronary a.
    digital subtraction a.
    femoral a.
    selective a.
**arteriohepatic dysplasia**
  **syndrome**
**arteriolar sclerosis**
**arteriole**
**arteriolith**
**arteriolitis**
    necrotizing a.
**arteriolonecrosis**
**arteriolosclerosis**
**arteriomalacia**
**arteriometer**
**arteriopalmus**

**arteriopathy**
  hypertensive a.
  plexogenic pulmonary a.
**arterioplania**
**arteriopressor**
**arteriorrhexis**
**arteriosclerosis**
  coronary a.
  hypertensive a.
  Mönckeberg's a.
  a. obliterans
  peripheral a.
**arteriosclerotic**
**arteriospasm**
**arteriosum**
  ligamentum a.
**arteriosus**
  conus a.
  ductus a.
  patent ductus a. (PDA)
  persistent ductus a.
  truncus a.
**arteriotomy**
  brachial a.
**arteriotony**
**arteriovenous (A-V, AV)**
  a. anastomosis
  a. aneurysm
  a. fistula
  a. malformation
  a. oxygen difference
  a. shunt
**arteritis**
  brachiocephalic a.
  cranial a.
  giant cell a.
  granulomatous a.
  Horton's a.
  mesenteric a.
  a. nodosa
  a. obliterans
  rheumatoid a.

  Takayasu's a.
  temporal a.
**artery, pl. arteries**
  aberrant a.
  accessory a.
  atrioventricular node a.
  axillary a.
  brachial a.
  brachiocephalic a.
  bronchial a.
  carotid a.
  celiac a.
  circumflex a.
  coarctation of
    pulmonary a.
  common carotid a.
  complete transposition
    of great arteries
  coronary a.
  diagonal a.
  d-transposition of great
    arteries (d-TGA)
  a. ectasia
  external carotid a.
  external mammary a.
  femoral a.
  first obtuse marginal a.
    (OM-1)
  gastroepiploic a.
  great a.
  iliac a.
  innominate a.
  internal carotid a.
  internal mammary a.
  intersegmental arteries
  intramural coronary
    arteries
  jejunal a.
  Kugel's a.
  left anterior
    descending a. (LAD)
  left circumflex a.
  left coronary a.

**artery** *(continued)*
    left internal
      mammary a. (LIMA)
    left main coronary a.
    malposition of great
      arteries (MGA)
    mammary a.
    marginal a.
    marginal arteries of
      Drummond
    parieto-occipital a.
    perineal a.
    peroneal a.
    popliteal a.
    posterior descending a.
      (PDA)
    posterior descending
      coronary a.
    profunda femoris a.
    pulmonary a. (PA)
    radial a.
    ramus intermedius a.
    renal a.
    retinal a.
    right coronary a. (RCA)
    right pulmonary a.
      (RPA)
    second obtuse
      marginal a. (OM-2)
    septal a.
    septal perforating
      arteries
    sinoatrial node a.
    sinus node a.
    subclavian a.
    superior carotid a.
    superior thyroid a.
    tibial a.
    transposition of great
      arteries
    ulnar a.
    umbilical a.
**arthritis**, pl. **arthritides**
    acute rheumatic a.

    juvenile rheumatoid a.
    rheumatoid a.
**arthritis-associated aortitis**
**arthropod venom**
**artifact**
    beam width a.
    catheter impact a.
    catheter whip a.
    end-pressure a.
    flow a.
    reverberation a.
    side lobe a.
**artifactual bradycardia**
**artificial**
    a. heart
    a. pacemaker
    a. respiration
    a. valve
**Arvin**
**AS**
    ankylosing spondylitis
    aortic stenosis
**As**
    arsenic
**ASC**
    ASC Alpha balloon
    ASC RX perfusion
      balloon catheter
**ascending**
    a. aorta (AA)
    a. aortography
**Aschner-Dagnini reflex**
**Aschner's**
    A. phenomenon
    A. reflex
**Aschoff**
    A. bodies
    A. nodule
**ascites**
    a. praecox
**ascorbic acid**
**ASD**
    atrial septal defect
**asequence**

**Ashley's phenomenon**
**Ashman's phenomenon**
**Ask-Upmark**
    A.-U. kidney
    A.-U. syndrome
**ASO**
    antistreptolysin O
**aspartate aminotransferase (AST)**
**aspergillosis**
*Aspergillus*
**asphygmia**
**asphyxia**
    cyanotic a.
    local a.
    symmetric a.
    traumatic a.
**aspirated and flushed**
**aspiration**
    fluid a.
**aspirin**
    buffered a.
    enteric-coated a.
**asplenia**
**assay**
**assessment**
    anatomic a.
    angiographic a.
    cardiovascular
      function a.
    causality a.
    echocardiographic a.
    functional a.
    hemodynamic a.
    invasive a.
    noninvasive a.
    postoperative a.
    transposition a.
**assisted ventilation**
**AST**
    aspartate aminotransferase
**asthenia**
    neurocirculatory a.
    vasoregulatory a.

**asthma**
    bronchial a.
    cardiac a.
**Astra pacemaker**
**ASTZ**
    antistreptozyme
    ASTZ test
**asymmetric**
    a. hypertrophy
    a. septal hypertrophy
**asymptomatic patient**
**asynchronous**
    a. pacing
    a. pulse generator
**asynchrony**
**asynergy**
**asystole**
    atrial a.
**asystolia**
**asystolic arrest**
**AT**
    atrial tachycardia
**A-T antiembolism stockings**
**ataxia**
    a. cordis
    Friedreich's a.
    hereditary a.
    spinocerebellar a.
**atenolol**
**atherectomy**
    a. catheter
    coronary a.
    directional coronary a.
    (DCA)
    a. index
**atheroblation laser**
**AtheroCath**
    Simpson A.
**atheroembolism**
**atherogenesis**
    monoclonal theory of a.
    response-to-injury
      hypothesis of a.
**atherogenic**

**atherolytic reperfusion guide wire**
**atheroma embolism**
**atheromatous**
    a. embolism
    a. plaque
**atherosclerosis**
    coronary a.
    coronary artery a.
    encrustation theory of a.
    lipogenic theory of a.
    a. obliterans
    premature a.
**atherosclerotic**
    a. aneurysm
    a. aortic disease
    a. aortography
    a. disease
    a. narrowing
    a. plaque
**atherosis**
**atherothrombosis**
**atherothrombotic**
**athlete's heart**
**athletic heart**
**AT-III**
    antithrombin III
**Ativan**
**ATP**
    antitachycardia pacemaker
    adenosine triphosphate
**ATPase**
    adenosinetriphosphatase
**AtPP**
    activated partial
    thromboplastin time
**ATRAC-II double-balloon catheter**
**ATRAC multipurpose balloon catheter**
**atracurium**
**atresia**
    aortic a.
    biliary a.

    mitral a.
    pulmonary a.
    pulmonic a.
    tricuspid a.
**atria**
**atrial**
    a. appendage
    a. arrhythmia
    a. asynchronous pacemaker
    a. asystole
    a. bigeminy
    a. capture
    a. capture threshold
    a. chaotic tachycardia
    a. complex
    a. demand pacemaker
    a. dissociation
    a. echo
    a. extrastimulus method
    a. extrasystole
    a. fibrillation
    a. fibrillation flutter
    a. flutter
    a. fusion beat
    a. gallop
    a. infarction
    a. kick
    a. lead impedance
    a. myocardial infarction
    a. myxoma
    a. natriuretic factor (ANF)
    a. natriuretic peptide
    a. pacing
    a. pacing stress test
    a. pacing study
    a. premature beat (APB)
    a. premature complexes (APC)
    a. premature contraction
    a. premature depolarizations
    a. pressure

a. pulse amplitude
a. pulsewidth
a. refractory period
a. rhythm
a. sensing configuration
a. sensitivity
a. septal aneurysm
a. septal defect (ASD)
a. septal defect single
disk closure device
a. septal defect umbrella
a. septectomy
a. septostomy
a. septum
a. sound
a. standstill
a. synchronous
pacemaker
a. synchronous pulse
generator
a. synchronous
ventricular inhibited
pacemaker
a. synchrony
a. systole
a. tachycardia (AT)
a. thrombus
a. transport function
a. triggered pulse
generator
**atrial-well technique**
**Atricor pacemaker**
**atriocarotid interval**
**atriohisian**
a. fibers
a. tract
**atrio-Hisian interval**
**atriopulmonary shunt**
**atrioseptal defect**
**atrioseptostomy**
balloon a.
**atriosystolic murmur**
**atrioventricular (A-V, AV)**

a. block
a. bundle
a. canal
a. canal defect
a. concordance
a. conduction
a. conduction
abnormality
a. connection anomaly
a. discordance
a. dissociation
a. extrasystole
a. flow rumbling
murmur
a. gradient
a. junction
a. junctional escape beat
a. junctional
reciprocating
tachycardia
a. junctional rhythm
a. junctional tachycardia
a. junction motion
a. nodal bigeminy
a. nodal extrasystole
a. nodal reentrant
tachycardia
a. nodal reentry
a. nodal rhythm
a. nodal tachycardia
a. node (AVN)
a. node artery
a. reciprocating
tachycardia
a. septal defect
a. sequential pacemaker
a. sulcus
a. valve
a. valve insufficiency
**atrioventricularis**
crus dextrum fasciculi a.
crus sinistrum
fasciculi a.

**atrioventriculosis**
  nodus a.
**atrium,** pl. **atria**
  accessory a.
  congenital single a.
  left a.
  right a.
  single a.
  a. thoracic catheter
**Atromid-S**
**atrophic**
  a. papulosis
  a. thrombosis
**atrophy**
  brown a.
  cyanotic a. of liver
  Erb's a.
  multiple system a.
  olivopontocerebellar a.
  optic a.
  peroneal muscular a.
  red a.
  spinal muscular a.
**atropine**
  a. test
**attack**
  anxiety a.
  heart a.
  transient ischemic a.
   (TIA)
  vagal a.
  vasovagal a.
**attenuation**
**attenuator**
**atypical**
  a. chest pain
  a. tamponade
  a. verrucous endocarditis
**Au**
  gold
**auditory alternans**
**Auenbrugger's sign**
**aureomycin**
  a. sensitivity

*aureus*
  *Staphylococcus a.*
**auricular**
  a. appendage
  a. appendectomy
  a. complex
  a. extrasystole
  a. fibrillation
  a. flutter
  a. standstill
  a. systole
  a. tachycardia
**auriculopressor reflex**
**auscultation**
  cardiac a.
**auscultatory**
  a. alternans
  a. gap
  a. sign
**Austin Flint murmur**
**Australian Therapeutic Trial**
**Austrian's syndrome**
**autogenous**
**autograft**
**autohypnosis**
**autoimmune disorder**
**autologous**
**automated edge detection**
**automatic**
  a. beat
  a. contraction
  a. exposure system
  a. implantable
   cardioverter-defibrillator
   (AICD)
  a. implantable
   defibrillator
  a. intracardiac
   defibrillator
  a. pacemaker
  a. ventricular
   contraction
**autonomic nervous system**

**autoregulation**
    heterometric a.
    homeometric a.
**autosome**
**Autostat ligating and**
  **hemostatic clips**
**auxocardia**
**A-V, AV**
  arteriovenous
  atrioventricular
    A-V block
    A-V conduction
    A-V dissociation
    A-V extrasystole
    A-V interval
    A-V nodal bigeminy
    A-V nodal extrasystole
    A-V nodal rhythm
    A-V nodal tachycardia
**average**
    a. mean pressure (AMP)
    a. pulse magnitude
**averaging**
    digital a.
    signal a.
**AVG**
  peak transaortic valve
  gradient
*avium*
    *Mycobacterium a.*
**AVN**
  atrioventricular node
**AVR**
  aortic valve replacement

**avulsion**
**A wave**
    precordial A w.
**axes**
**axial control**
**axillary**
    a. artery
    a. artery occlusion
    a. vein
    a. vein occlusion
**Axios 04 pacemaker**
**axis, pl. axes**
    a. deviation
    electrical a.
    instantaneous
     electrical a.
    long a. (LAX)
    mean electrical a.
    normal a.
    a. shift
    short a. (SAX)
**Ayerza's**
    A. disease
    A. syndrome
**azapetine phosphate**
**azathioprine**
**azotemia**
    extrarenal a.
    postrenal a.
    prerenal a.
    renal a.
**azygos vein**

B

baby
  blue b.
Bachmann's bundle
Bacille bilié de Calmette-
  Guérin (BCG)
bacillus
  Löffler's b.
backbleed
backbleeding
backward heart failure
bacteremia
bacteria
bacteria-free stage of bacterial
  endocarditis
bacterial
  b. endocarditis
  b. infection
  b. myocarditis
  b. pericarditis
bactericidal titer
*Bacteroides oralis*
baffle
  interatrial b.
  intra-atrial b.
  Mustard interatrial b.
  Senning intra-atrial b.
bag
  Douglas b.
  Sones hemostatic b.
  Voorhees b.
bailout catheter
Baim catheter
Bainbridge
  B. effect
  B. reflex
BAL
  bronchoalveolar lavage
Balectrode pacing catheter
Balke protocol
Balke-Ware
  B.-W. protocol
  B.-W. test

ball
  b. thrombus
  b. valve
  b. variance
ball-cage valve
ballerina-foot pattern
ballet
  cardiac b.
ball-in-cage prosthetic valve
ballistocardiogram
ballistocardiograph (BCG)
ballistocardiography
balloon
  b. angioplasty
  b. angioplasty catheter
  b. aortic valvotomy
  b. aortic valvuloplasty
  Arrow Berman
   angiographic b.
  ASC Alpha b.
  b. atrial septostomy
  b. atrial septotomy
  b. atrioseptostomy
  Baxter Intrepid b.
  bifoil b.
  b. catheter
  b. coarctation
   angioplasty
  Cribier-Letac b.
  Cribier-Letac aortic
   valvuloplasty b.
  Datascope b.
  b. dilation
  b. flotation catheter
  hadow b.
  b. inflation
  Inoue b.
  Inoue self-guiding b.
  intra-aortic b.
  Kay b.
  Kontron b.
  b. laser angioplasty

**balloon** *(continued)*
    latex b.
    Mansfield b.
    b. mitral valvotomy
      (BMV)
    b. mitral valvuloplasty
    NoProfile b.
    b. occlusion
    Olbert b.
    Owens b.
    polyethylene b.
    polyvinyl chloride b.
    b. pulmonary valvotomy
    b. pulmonary
      valvuloplasty (BPV)
    b. pump
    b. rupture
    b. septostomy
    sizing b.
    Slinky b.
    Thruflex b.
    trefoil b.
    b. tricuspid valvotomy
    b. valvotomy
    b. valvuloplasty
    b. valvuloplasty catheter
**balloon-centered argon laser**
**balloon-expandable stent**
**ballooning mitral cusp**
  **syndrome**
**balloon-occlusion pulmonary**
  **angiography**
**balloon-tip catheter**
**balloon-tipped**
    b.-t. flow-directed
      catheter
    b.-t. thermodilution
      catheter
**Balloon Valvuloplasty Registry**
**ball-valve thrombus**
**Bamberger's sign**
**band**
    contraction b.
    moderator b.

    pulmonary artery b.'s
    b. saw effect
    Z b.
**Baratol**
**barbed hook**
**barbiturate**
**Bard**
    B. clamshell septal
      umbrella
    B. electrophysiology
      catheter
    B. PDA umbrella
    B. percutaneous
      cardiopulmonary
      support system
**Bard-Parker blade**
**barium enema**
**Barlow syndrome**
**barometric pressure**
**baroreceptor**
    cardiac b.
**baroreflex**
**Barrett's esophagus**
**barrier**
    blood-brain b.
    blood-retina b.
    placental b.
**baseline**
    b. fetal heart rate
    b. variability of fetal
      heart rate
**baseplate**
    winged b.
**basic fibroblastic growth**
  **factor (BFGF)**
**basilic vein**
**basket**
    Medi-Tech
      multipurpose b.
    b. retrieval catheter
**bath**
    film fixer b.
    film wash b.
    fixer b.

*Ultrathin
Tyshak
maxxum*

Nauheim b.
wash b.
**bathycardia**
**battery**
Celsa b.
lithium b.
nickel-cadmium b.
**Bauer's syndrome**
**Baumès symptom**
**Baxter**
B. angioplasty catheter
B. Intrepid balloon
**Bayes' theorem**
**BAY k 8644**
**Bayliss theory**
**Baypress**
**Bazett's formula**
**BBB**
bundle branch block
**BBBB**
bilateral bundle branch
block
**B-cell**
B-c. antibody
B-c. pymphoma
**BCG**
Bacille bilié de Calmette-
Guérin
ballistocardiograph
**Beall scissors**
**beam width artifact**
**beat**
apex b.
atrial fusion b.
atrial premature b.
(APB)
atrioventricular
junctional escape b.
automatic b.
capture b.
combination b.
coupled b.
dependent b.
Dressler b.

dropped b.
echo b.
ectopic b.
escape b., escaped b.
fascicular b.
forced b.
fusion b.
heart b.
interference b.
junctional b.
junctional escape b.
mixed b.
paired b.
parasystolic b.
b.'s per minute (bpm)
premature b.
premature atrial b.
premature junctional b.
premature ventricular b.
(PVB)
pseudofusion b.
reciprocal b.
retrograde b.
summation b.
ventricular fusion b.
ventricular premature b.
(VPB)
**beat-to-beat variation of fetal**
**heart rate**
**Beaver blade**
**Becker**
B. dystrophy
B.-type tardive muscular
dystrophy
**Becker's disease**
**Beck miniature aortic clamp**
**Beck's triad**
**Becton-Dickinson guide wire**
**beef insulin**
**beer-drinker's cardiomyopathy**
**beer heart**
**Beer-Lambert principle**
**bee venom**

Bental
procedure

**behavior**
   type A b.
   type B b.
**behavioral**
   b. factor
   b. therapy
**Behçet's**
   B. disease
   B. syndrome
**Bellavar medical support stockings**
**bellows murmur**
**Benadryl**
**benazapril**
**Bendrofluazide**
**bendroflumethiazide**
**benign hypertension**
**Bentson exchange straight guide wire**
**benzathine benzyl penicillin**
**benzodiazepine**
**benzothiadiazide**
**benzthiazide**
**bepridil HCl**
**Bergmeister's papilla**
**beriberi**
   cerebral b.
   dry b.
   infantile b.
   wet b.
**Berman**
   B. angiographic catheter
   B. balloon flotation catheter
   B. catheter
**Bernheim's syndrome**
**Bernoulli's theorem**
**Bernstein test**
**beta**
   b. agonist
   b. blocker
   b. blocking agent
   b. lipoprotein
   b. ray

   b. receptor
   b. thromboglobulin
**beta-adrenoreceptor**
   b.-a. agonist
   b.-a. blocker
**Betaloc**
**betaxolol**
**bethanechol chloride**
**bethanidine**
**Beuren syndrome**
**bevantolol**
**bezafibrate**
**Bezalip**
**Bezold-Jarisch reflex**
**BFGF**
   basic fibroblastic growth factor
**B-H interval**
**Bi**
   bismuth
**bicarbonate**
   sodium b.
**bicarbonaturia**
**bicardiogram**
**bicuspid aortic valve**
**bicuspidization**
**bicycle ergometry**
**bidirectional**
   b. shunt
   b. shunt calculation
   b. ventricular tachycardia
**Bier block anesthesia**
**bifascicular**
   b. block
   b. heart block
**bifid P-waves**
**bifoil**
   b. balloon
   b. catheter
**bifurcation**
   b. of aorta
   carotid b.
   coronary b.

b. of pulmonary trunk
b. of trachea
**bigemina**
**bigeminal**
    b. pulse
    b. rhythm
**bigeminus**
    pulsus b.
**bigeminy**
    atrial b.
    atrioventricular nodal b.,
      A-V nodal b.
    escape-capture b.
    nodal b.
    reciprocal b.
    ventricular b.
**bilateral**
    b. adrenal hyperplasia
    b. bundle branch block
      (BBBB)
**bile**
    b. acid binding resin
    b. acid sequestrant
**biliary**
    b. atresia
    b. colic
    b. disease
**billowing mitral valve**
  **syndrome**
**bimanual precordial palpation**
**Bing stylet**
**Binswanger's disease**
**bioavailability**
**biocompatibility**
**bioelectric current**
**bioelectricity**
**biological**
    b. fitness
    b. half-life
**bioprosthesis**
    Carpentier-Edwards b.
**bioprosthetic valve**
**biopsy**
    catheter-guided b.

endomyocardial b.
b. forceps
lung b.
pericardial b.
ventricular b.
**bioptome**
    Caves-Schultz b.
    Cordis b.
    Kawai b.
    King b.
    Konno b.
    Mansfield b.
    Olympus b.
    Stanford b.
**Biotronik**
    B. lead connector
    B. pacemaker
**biperiden**
**biplane**
    b. aortography
    b. fluoroscopy
    b. formula
    imaging b.
    b. ventriculography
**bipolar**
    b. lead
    b. myocardial electrode
    b. pacemaker
**biprosthetic prosthetic valve**
**birds-eye catheter**
**Bird's Nest vena caval filter**
**bisferious**
    b. pulse
**Bishop's sphygmoscope**
**bishydroxycoumarin**
**bismuth (Bi)**
**bisoprolol**
**BIVAD centrifugal left and**
  **right device**
**biventricular endomyocardial**
  **fibrosis**
**Björk method of Fontan**
  **procedure**

**Björk-Shiley**
   B.-S. heart valve holder
   B.-S. heart valve sizer
   B.-S. prosthetic valve
   B.-S. valve
**b knuckle**
**blackout**
   shallow water b.
**black widow spider venom**
**blade**
   b. atrial septostomy
   Bard-parker b.
   Beaver b.
   b. control wire holder
   b. septostomy
   b. septostomy catheter
**Blalock-Hanlon**
   B.-H. atrial septectomy
   B.-H. operation
**Blalock-Taussig**
   B.-T. operation
   B.-T. procedure
   B.-T. shunt
**bland embolism**
**Bland-White-Garland syndrome**
*Blastomyces dermatitidis*
**blastomycosis**
**bloater**
   blue b.'s
**Blocadren**
**block**
   anterograde b.
   arborization b.
   atrioventricular b., A-
      V b.
   bifascicular b.
   bifascicular heart b.
   bundle branch b. (BBB)
   complete A-V b.
   complete heart b.
   conduction b.
   congenital heart b.
   divisional b.
   divisional heart b.

   entrance b.
   exit b.
   fascicular b.
   fascicular heart b.
   first degree A-V b.
   first degree heart b.
   focal b.
   heart b.
   intra-atrial b.
   intraventricular b., I-
      V b.
   left bundle branch b.
      (LBBB)
   Mobitz b.
   Mobitz
      atrioventricular b.
   Mobitz type I
      atrioventricular b.
   Mobitz type II
      atrioventricular b.
   Mobitz types of
      atrioventricular b.
   peri-infarction b.
   protective b.
   retrograde b.
   right bundle branch b.
      (RBBB)
   second degree A-V b.
   second degree heart b.
   sinoatrial b.,
      sinoauricular b.,
      sinus b.
   sinoatrial exit b.
   suprahisian b.
   third degree heart b.
   transient heart b.
   unidirectional b.
   Wenckebach
      atrioventricular b.
   Wilson b.
**β-blockade**
**blocker**
   adrenoceptor b.
   alpha-adrenergic b.

alpha-adrenoreceptor b.
beta b.
beta-adrenoreceptor b.
calcium channel b.
ganglionic b.
renin-angiotensin b.
slow channel b.

**blood**
b. clot
b. count
b. dyscrasia
b. flow
b. flow measurement
b. gases
mixed venous b.
b. oxygen levels
b. pool imaging
b. pressure (BP)
b. pressure cuff
b. sampling
b. test
b. viscosity
b. volume
b. volume distribution

**blood-brain barrier**
**bloodless phlebotomy**
**bloodletting**
**blood-retina barrier**
**bloodstream**
**blowing murmur**
**blue**
b. baby
b. bloaters
b. sclera
b. toe syndrome

**blunt**
b. eversion
b. eversion carotid
endarterectomy
b. injury
b. trauma

**BMI**, gen. **indicis**, pl. **indices**,
**indexes**
body mass index

**B-mode echocardiography**
**BMV**
balloon mitral valvotomy
**body**
Aschoff b.'s
central fibrous b.
b. fat
fibrous b.
foreign b.
b. mass index (BMI)
b. position
b. surface area (BSA)
b. surface mapping
**bolometer**
**bolus injection**
**bond**
soldered b.
**bone**
fibrous dysplasia of b.
b. marrow
transplantation
Paget's disease of b.
**bony heart**
**boot-shaped heart**
**bootstrap**
b. dilation
b. two-vessel angioplasty
b. two-vessel technique
**borderline hypertension**
**Borg scale**
**Borst side-arm introducer set**
**Bouillaud's disease**
**Bourassa catheter**
*bovis*
*Mycobacterium b.*
**Bowditch's**
B. law
B. phenomenon
**box**
Elecath switch b.
**BP**
blood pressure
British Pharmacopoeia

**bpm**
>  beats per minute

**BPV**
>  balloon pulmonary
>  valvuloplasty

**brachial**
>  b. approach
>  b. arteriotomy
>  b. artery
>  b. artery approach
>  b. artery cutdown
>  b. artery thrombosis
>  b. catheter
>  b. pulse
>  b. vein

**brachial/ankle index**

**brachiocephalic**
>  b. arteritis
>  b. artery
>  b. ischemia
>  b. system
>  b. vein

**brachiogram**

**Bracht-Wachter lesion**

**brachycardia**

**Bradbury-Eggleston syndrome**

**Bradilan**

**bradyarrhythmia**

**bradyarrhythmic arrest**

**bradycardia**
>  artifactual b.
>  cardiomuscular b.
>  central b.
>  essential b.
>  fetal b.
>  idiopathic b.
>  nodal b.
>  postinfectious b.
>  sinus b.
>  ventricular b.

**bradycardia-dependent aberrancy**

**bradycardia-tachycardia syndrome**

**bradycardic**

**bradycrotic**

**bradydiastole**

**bradykinin**

**bradyrhythmia**

**bradysphygmia**

**brain**
>  b. abscess
>  b. aneurysm
>  b. death
>  b. infarct
>  b. murmur

**branch**
>  b. lesion
>  b. pulmonary artery
>  stenosis
>  b. vessel occlusion

**Branham's sign**

**Braunwald-Cutter**
>  B.-C. prosthetic valve
>  B.-C. valve

**bread-and-butter pericardium**

**breakaway splice**

**breast pang**

**breath-holding test**

**breathing**
>  intermittent positive
>  pressure b. (IPPB)

**bregmocardiac reflex**

**bretylium**
>  b. tosylate

**Bretylol**

**Brevibloc**

**Brevital**

**bridge**
>  muscle b.
>  myocardial b.
>  Wheatstone b.

**bridging**
>  myocardial b.

**Bright's disease**

**British Pharmacopoeia (BP)**

**Broadbent's sign**

**Brockenbrough**
- B. catheter
- B. curved needle
- B. curved-tip occluder
- B. needle
- B. sign
- B. transseptal catheter

**Brockenbrough-Braunwald sign**
**Brock's procedure**
**bromide**
- pancuronium b.

**bromocriptine**
**bronchi**
**bronchial**
- b. artery
- b. asthma
- b. collateral
- b. collateral artery murmur

**bronchiectasis**
**bronchitis**
- winter b.

**bronchoalveolar lavage (BAL)**
**bronchodilator**
**bronchospasm**
**bronchus**, pl. **bronchi**
**brown**
- b. atrophy
- b. induration of lung

**Bruce**
- B. protocol
- B. treadmill protocol

*Brucella*
**brucellosis**
**bruit**
- abdominal b.
- aneurysmal b.
- carotid b.
- b. de canon
- b. de diable
- b. de galop
- b. de lime
- b. de moulin
- b. de rappel
- b. de Roger
- b. de scie ou de rape
- b. de soufflet
- b. de tabourka
- b. de triolet
- thyroid b.
- Traube's b.

**Brushfield's spot**
**Bryant's ampulla**
**Bryant mitral hook**
**BSA**
- body surface area

**BTF-37 arterial blood filter**
**bucardia**
*buccalis*
- *Leptotrichia* b.

**bucindolol**
**buckled aorta**
**buckling**
- midsystolic b.

**Budd-Chiari syndrome**
**Buerger's disease**
**buffered aspirin**
**Bufferin**
**bulbar pulse**
**bulboventricular**
- b. fold
- b. foramen
- b. groove
- b. loop
- b. sulcus
- b. tube

**bulbus cordis**
**bulldog clamp**
**bullet wound**
**bull's-eye plot**
**bull's eye polar coordinate mapping**
**bumetanide**
**Bumex**
**bundle**
- atrioventricular b.
- Bachmann's b.
- b. branch block (BBB)

**bundle** *(continued)*
    b. branch reentrant
      tachycardia
    b. branch reentry
    His b.
    b. of His
    Keith's b.
    Kent's b.
**bundle branch block (BBB)**
    bilateral b. b. b.
      (BBBB)
    left b. b. b. (LBBB)
    right b. b. b. (RBBB)
**Bunnell-Howard arthrodesis**
  **clamp**
**bupivacaine**
**bur**
**Burinex**
*burnetii*
    *Coxiella b.*
**Buschke**
    scleredema of B.

**buttonhole**
    mitral b.
    b. stenosis
**buttress**
    Teflon pledget suture b.
**bypass**
    aortocoronary b.
    aortofemoral b.
    aortoiliac b.
    cardiopulmonary b.
      (CPB)
    coronary b.
    coronary artery b. graft
      (CABG)
    femorotibial b.
    b. graft
    b. graft catheter
    b. graft catheterization
    heart-lung b.
    b. surgery
    b. tract

**CA**
carcinoma
cardiac arrest
cancer
chronologic age
cytosine arabinoside
**CABG**
coronary artery bypass graft
**Cabot-Locke murmur**
**cachectic**
c. endocarditis
**cachexia**
**CAD**
coronary artery disease
**cadmium (Cd)**
**café-au-lait spot**
**café coronary**
**caffeine**
**caged-ball valve**
**c-a interval**
**Calan**
**calcific**
c. debris
c. mitral stenosis
c. nodular aortic
stenosis
c. pericarditis
**calcification**
arterial c.
pericardial c.
valvular c.
**calcified nodule**
**calcinosis**
**calcium**
c. antagonist
c. channel
c. channel agonist
c. channel antagonists
c. channel blocker
c. channel blocking
agent

c. chloride
fluoroscopic c.
c. gluconate
c. ion
c. oxalate
c. oxalate deposition
c. paradox
c. rigor
c. sign
c. transient
*calcoaceticus*
*Acinetobacter c.*
**calculation**
bidirectional shunt c.
**calculus**, gen. and pl. **calculi**
cardiac c.
**calibration**
**calibrator**
Fogarty c.
**Calman**
C. carotid clamp
C. ring clamp
**calmodulin**
**camera**
Anger c.
Anger scintillation c.
cine c.
gamma c.
scintillation c.
video c.
**cAMP**
cyclic adenosine
monophosphate
*Campylobacter*
**camsylate**
trimetaphan c.
**Canadian**
C. Cardiovascular
Society
C. Cardiovascular
Society classification

**Canadian** *(continued)*
    C. Cardiovascular
      Society grading of
      angina
**canal**
    atrioventricular c.
    persistent
      atrioventricular c.
**cancer (CA)**
*Candida*
**candidiasis**
**candoxatril**
*canis*
    *Toxocara c.*
**cannon**
    c. sound
    c. a wave
    c. wave
**cannonball pulse**
**Cannon's**
    C. formula
    C. theory
**cannula**
    aortic perfusion c.
    cardiovascular c.
    Churchill cardiac
      suction c.
    Cobe small vessel c.
    femoral perfusion c.
    Grüntzig femoral
      stiffening c.
    Razi c. introducer
    saphenous vein c.
    Tibbs arterial c.
    vein graft c.
    vena cava c.
    venous c.
**cannulation**
**canola oil**
**canrenoate potassium**
**canrenone**
**cantering rhythm**
**Cantrell's pentalogy**

**capacitance vessel**
**capacitor forming time**
**capacity**
    aerobic c.
    diffusing c.
    exercise c.
    oxygen carrying c.
    vital c.
    work c.
**capillaropathy**
**capillary,** pl. **capillaries**
    c. pressure
    c. pulse
**Capiscint**
**Capoten**
**Capozide**
**caprizant**
**captopril**
**capture**
    atrial c.
    c. beat
    ventricular c.
**Carabello's sign**
**carbamazepine**
**Carbocaine**
**carbohydrate intolerance**
**Carbomedics cardiac valve**
  **prosthesis**
**carbomethoxyisopropyl**
  **isonitrile**
**carbon**
    c. dioxide
    c. dioxide production
    c. dioxide tension
    c. disulfide
    c. monoxide
**carbon-11**
**carbonic anhydrase inhibitor**
**carcinoid**
    c. heart disease
    c. murmur
    c. plaque
    c. syndrome

c. tumor
c. valve disease
**carcinoma (CA)**
**Cardabid**
**Cardak percutaneous catheter introducer**
**Cardene**
**cardiac**
  c. accident
  c. amyloidosis
  c. aneurysm
  c. apex
  c. arrest (CA)
  c. arrhythmia
  c. arrhythmia suppression trial (CAST)
  c. asthma
  c. auscultation
  c. ballet
  c. baroreceptor
  c. calculus
  c. catheter
  c. catheterization
  c. cirrhosis
  c. competence
  c. compression
  c. conduction
  c. conduction system
  c. contraction
  c. contusion
  c. cycle
  c. death
  c. depressor reflex
  c. diastole
  direct c. puncture
  c. diuretic
  c. dysrhythmia
  c. edema
  c. enlargement
  c. enzyme
  c. examination
  c. failure
  c. function

c. glycogenosis
c. glycoside
c. hemoptysis
c. heterotaxia
c. hypertrophy
c. impulse
c. incompetence
c. index (CI)
c. infarction
c. insufficiency
c. ischemia
c. liver
c. lung
c. mapping
c. mass
c. massage
c. memory
c. metastasis
c. monitor
c. murmur
c. muscle
c. myosin
c. neurosis
c. output
c. output index
c. output measurement
c. perforation
c. performance
c. polyp
c. rehabilitation
c. reserve
c. resuscitation
c. rhythm
c. risk index
c. rupture
c. sarcoma
c. sensory nerve
c. silhouette
c. souffle
c. sound
c. standstill
c. status
c. surgery
c. symphysis

cardiac *(continued)*
    c. tamponade
    c. telemetry
    c. transplantation
    c. tumor
    c. valve
    c. valve prosthesis
    c. vein
    c. volume
    c. wall thickening
cardialgia
cardiataxia
cardiatelia
cardiectasia
cardiectopia
Cardilate
cardinal vein
cardioaccelerator
cardioactive
cardioangiography
cardioarterial interval
*Cardiobacterium hominis*
cardiocairograph
cardiocele
cardiocentesis
cardiochalasia
cardioclasia
cardiodynamics
cardiodynia
cardiofacial syndrome
cardiogenesis
cardiogenic
    c. pulmonary edema
    c. shock
cardiogram
    apex c.
    esophageal c.
    vector c.
cardiograph
cardiography
    apex c.
    Doppler c.
    echo-Doppler c.

    ultrasound c.
    vector c.
Cardio-Green
cardiohemothrombus
cardiohepatomegaly
cardioinhibitory type
cardiokinetic
cardiokymogram
cardiokymograph
cardiokymography
Cardiolite
cardiolith
cardiologist
cardiology
cardiolysis
cardiomalacia
cardiomegaly
    glycogen c.
    idiopathic c.
Cardiometrics cardiotomy
    reservoir
cardiometry
cardiomotility
cardiomuscular bradycardia
cardiomyoliposis
cardiomyopathy
    African c.
    alcoholic c.
    beer-drinker's c.
    cobalt c.
    congestive c.
    diabetic c.
    dilated c.
    doxorubicin c.
    familial hypertrophic
        obstructive c.
    fibroplastic c.
    genetic hypertrophic c.
    HIV c.
    hypertensive
        hypertrophic c.
    hypertrophic c.
    hypertrophic
        obstructive c.

idiopathic c.
idiopathic dilated c.
idiopathic restrictive c.
infiltrative c.
ischemic c.
nephropathic c.
obliterative c.
obstructive
hypertrophic c.
pediatric c.
postpartum c.
primary c.
rejection c.
restrictive c.
secondary c.
**cardioneural**
**cardioneuropathy**
**cardioneurosis**
**cardio-omentopexy**
**cardiopaludism**
**cardiopathia nigra**
**cardiopathy**
**cardiopericardiopexy**
**cardiophobia**
**cardiophone**
**cardiophony**
**cardiophrenia**
**cardioplegia**
cold blood c.
c. cooling
normothermic c.
**cardioplegic**
**cardioptosia**
**cardiopulmonary**
c. arrest
c. bypass (CPB)
c. murmur
c. resuscitation (CPR)
c. support
**Cardioquin**
**cardiorespiratory murmur**
**cardiorrhaphy**
**cardiorrhexis**
**cardioschisis**

**cardioscope**
**cardioselectivity**
**cardiosphygmograph**
**cardiotachometer**
**CardioTec**
**cardiothoracic ratio**
**cardiothrombus**
**cardiothyrotoxicosis**
**cardiotomy reservoir**
**cardiotonic**
**cardiotoxicity**
Adriamycin c.
**cardiotoxic myolysis**
**cardiotoxin**
**cardiovalvotomy**
**cardiovalvulitis**
**cardiovalvulotomy**
**cardiovascular**
c. accident
c. cannula
c. clamp
c. collapse
c. disability
c. excitatory centers
c. fitness
c. function
c. function assessment
c. inhibitory centers
c. pressure
c. stylet
c. syphilis
c. system
**cardioversion**
direct-current c.
elective c.
electrical c.
**cardioverter**
**cardioverter-defibrillator**
automatic
implantable c.-d.
(AICD)
CPI PRX
implantable c.-d.
implantable c.-d.

41

**cardioverter-defibrillator**
*(continued)*
    Intermedics RES Q
     implantable c.-d.
    Medtronic PCD
     implantable c.-d.
    Siemens Siecure
     implantable c.-d.
    Telectronics ATP
     implantable c.-d.
    Ventritex Cadence
     implantable c.-d.
**cardiovirus**
**carditis**
    rheumatic c.
**Cardizem**
**Cardizem CD**
**Cardizem SR**
**Cardura**
**care**
    critical c.
    emergency c.
    intensive c.
    managed c.
**Carey Coombs murmur**
**Carfin**
**carinatum**
    pectus c.
**carneae**
    trabeculae c.
**carnitine**
**Carolon life support**
**antiembolism stockings**
**carotid**
    c. angiography
    c. artery
    c. artery murmur
    c. artery shunt
    c. bifurcation
    c. bruit
    c. Doppler
    c. endarterectomy
    c. pulse
    c. pulse tracing

    c. sheath
    c. shudder
    c. sinus
    c. sinus hypersensitivity
    c. sinus massage
    c. sinus nerve
    c. sinus reflex
    c. sinus syncope
    c. sinus syndrome
    c. stenosis
    c. upstroke
**carotid artery**
    common c. a.
    external c. a.
    internal c. a.
**carotid-cavernous fistula**
**carotodynia, carotidynia**
**Carpentier**
    C. rings
    C. stent
**Carpentier-Edwards**
    C.-E. bioprosthesis
    C.-E. valve
**carteolol**
**Carvallo's sign**
**carvedilol**
**CASS**
   Coronary Artery Surgery
   Study
**CAST**
   cardiac arrhythmia
   suppression trial
**Castroviejo needle holder**
**catacrotic pulse**
**catacrotism**
**catadicrotic pulse**
**catadicrotism**
**Catapres**
**Catapres CR**
**Catapres-TTS**
**catatricrotic**
**catatricrotism**
**catecholamine action**
**catenoid**

**catheter**
 c. ablation
 ACS angioplasty c.
 ACS balloon c.
 ACS RX coronary
  dilatation c.
 c. adapter
 AL II guiding c.
 Amplatz c.
 Amplatz coronary c.
 Amplatz high-flo torque
  control c.
 Angiocath c.
 Angioflow high-flow c.
 angiographic c.
 angioplasty guiding c.
 angled pigtail c.
 angulated
  multipurpose c.
 Arani c.
 Argyle c.
 Arrow balloon wedge c.
 Arrow-Howes c.
 arterial embolectomy c.
 c. arteriography
 ASC RX perfusion
  balloon c.
 atherectomy c.
 ATRAC-II double-
  balloon c.
 ATRAC multipurpose
  balloon c.
 atrium thoracic c.
 bailout c.
 Baim c.
 Balectrode pacing c.
 balloon c.
 balloon angioplasty c.
 balloon flotation c.
 balloon-tip c.
 balloon-tipped flow-
  directed c.
 balloon-tipped
  thermodilution c.

 balloon valvuloplasty c.
 Bard electrophysiology c.
 basket retrieval c.
 Baxter angioplasty c.
 Berman c.
 Berman angiographic c.
 Berman balloon
  flotation c.
 bifoil c.
 birds-eye c.
 blade septostomy c.
 Bourassa c.
 brachial c.
 Brockenbrough c.
 Brockenbrough
  transseptal c.
 bypass graft c.
 cardiac c.
 central venous c.
 Clark expanding
  mesh c.
 Clark helix c.
 Clark rotating cutter c.
 conductance c.
 Cordis c.
 coronary angiographic c.
 coronary seeking c.
 Cournand c.
 Cournand quadpolar c.
 Cribier-Letac c.
 Critikon balloon
  temporary pacing c.
 Critikon balloon wedge
  pressure c.
 Cynosar c.
 Dacron c.
 Deseret flow-directed
  thermodilution c.
 Doppler c.
 double-balloon c.
 double-lumen c.
 drill-tip c.
 Ducor c.
 Edwards c.

**catheter** *(continued)*
electrode c.
El Gamal coronary
bypass c.
c. embolectomy
embolectomy c.
c. embolus
Encapsulon epidural c.
end-hole #7 French c.
Eppendorf c.
FAST right heart
cardiovascular c.
fiberoptic c.
fiber optic c. delivery
system
fiberoptic oximeter c.
flow-directed c.
flow-directed balloon
cardiovascular c.
fluid-filled c.
Fogarty c.
Fogarty embolectomy c.
c. fragment
French double lumen c.
French JR4 Schneider c.
French SAL c.
French shaft c.
French sizing of c.
Gensini c.
Gensini coronary
arteriography c.
Goodale-Lubin c.
Gorlin c.
Grollman c.
Grollman pulmonary
artery seeking c.
Grüntzig c.
c. guide holder
c. guide wire
guiding c.
Hakko Dwelicath c.
Hancock embolectomy c.
Hancock fiberoptic c.

Hancock hydrogen
detection c.
Hancock luminal
electrophysiologic
recording c.
Hancock wedge-
pressure c.
Hartzler balloon c.
Hartzler dilatation c.
head-hunter c.
Helix PTCA
dilatation c.
high-flow c.
c. holder
c. hub
c. impact artifact
impedance c.
Inoue balloon c.
c. instability
Intimax vascular c.
intra-aortic balloon c.
intracardiac c.
Intrepid balloon c.
c. introduction method
Josephson c.
Josephson quadpolar c.
Jostra c.
JR4 c.
JR5 c.
Judkins c.
Judkins coronary c.
Judkins guiding c.
Judkins torque
control c.
Kensey c.
laserprobe c.
left coronary c.
left heart c.
Lehman c.
Lehman
ventriculography c.
Lo-Profile balloon c.
Lumelec pacing c.
c. manipulation

manometer tipped c.
Mansfield Atri-Pace I c.
Mansfield balloon c.
c. mapping
marker c.
Medi-Tech balloon c.
Medi-Tech steerable c.
memory c.
Micross dilatation c.
Mikro-Tip c.
Millar c.
monofoil c.
monometer-tipped c.
Mullins c.
multilayer design c.
multipurpose c.
multisensor c.
Mylar c.
Namic c.
Nestor guiding c.
NIH c.
NIH marking c.
nonflotation c.
non flow-directed c.
Norton flow-directed
  Swan-Ganz
  thermodilution c.
Novoste c.
Nycore-pigtail c.
optical fiber c.
Opticath oximeter c.
Owens c.
Owens balloon c.
Owens Lo-Profile
  dilatation c.
pacemaker c.
Pacewedge dual-pressure
  bipolar pacing c.
pacing c.
park blade
  septostomy c.
c. patency
pediatric pigtail c.

percutaneous rotational
  thrombectomy c.
Per-Q-Cath
  percutaneously inserted
  central venous c.
Picolino monorail c.
pigtail c.
preshaped c.
Procath
  electrophysiology c.
Profile Plus balloon
  dilatation c.
Pro-Flo c.
PWP monitoring c.
quadpolar w/Damato
  curve c.
radiopaque calibrated c.
Rashkind c.
Rashkind septostomy
  balloon c.
reperfusion c.
right coronary c.
right heart c.
Ritchie c.
Rodriguez c.
Rodriguez-Alvarez c.
Rotablator c.
rotational angioplasty c.
rotational dynamic
  angioplasty c.
Safe-T-Coat heparin-
  coated
  thermodilution c.
Schneider c.
Schoonmaker c.
Sci-Med angioplasty c.
self-guiding c.
self-positioning
  balloon c.
Shiley c.
Sidewinder percutaneous
  intra-aortic balloon c.
Simpson atherectomy c.

catheter *(continued)*

Simpson coronary AtheroCath c.
Skinny balloon c.
Slinky balloon c.
Slinky PTCA c.
Smart position-sensing c.
Sones c.
Sones coronary c.
Sorenson thermodilution c.
Stertzer brachial c.
Stertzer guiding c.
Swan-Ganz c.
Swan-Ganz bipolar pacing c.
c. system
thermodilution c.
thermodilution balloon c.
c. tip occluder
Torktherm torque control c.
torque control balloon c.
Tracker soft stream side hole microinfusion c.
transluminal angioplasty c.
transluminal extraction c.
transluminal extraction-endarterectomy c. (TEC)
transseptal c.
trefoil c.
trefoil balloon c.
tripolar w/Damato curve c.
Uniweave c.
Uresil embolectomy thrombectomy c.
urinary c.
USCI c.

vascular access c.
velocity c. technique
ventriculographic c.
V. Mueller c.
wedge pressure balloon c.
Wexler c.
c. whip
c. whip artifact
Zucker c.
Zucker multi-purpose bipolar c.

**catheter-guided biopsy**
**catheter-induced spasm**
**catheterization**

bypass graft c.
cardiac c.
combined heart c.
c. complications
coronary sinus c.
hepatic vein c.
interventional c.
interventional cardiac c.
Judkins-Sones technique of cardiac c.
left heart c.
outpatient c.
pulmonary artery c.
retrograde c.
right heart c.
routine right heart c.
c. technique
transseptal c.
transseptal left heart c.

**catheter-related peripheral vessel spasm**
**catheter-snare system**
**catheter-tip**

c.-t. micromanometer system
c.-t. spasm

**Cath-Lok catheter locking device**
**causality assessment**

**cava**
> inferior vena c. (IVC)
> superior vena c. (SVC)
> vena c.

**CAVB**
> complete atrioventricular block

**Caves-Schultz bioptome**
**cavitation**
**cavitis**
**cavus**
> pes c.

**CBC**
> complete blood count

**CBF**
> cerebral blood flow
> coronary blood flow

**CB lead**
**CCS endocardial pacing lead**
**CCU**
> coronary care unit

**Cd**
> cadmium

**C to E amplitude**
**Cedilanid-D**
**ceftriaxone**
**celiac artery**
**celiprolol**
**cell**
> ameboid c.
> foam c.
> lepidic c.
> c. membrane
> N c.
> P c.
> Purkinje c.'s
> smooth-muscle c.
> T c.
> transitional c.

**Cell Saver**
**cellular embolism**
**celophlebitis**
**Celsa battery**

**center**
> cardiovascular excitatory c.'s
> cardiovascular inhibitory c.'s

**centerline method of wall motion analysis**
**CentoRx**
**central**
> c. approach
> c. bradycardia
> c. core wire
> c. fibrous body
> c. terminal electrode
> c. venous catheter
> c. venous line
> c. venous pressure (CVP)

**centronuclear myopathy**
**Centyl**
**cephalic vein**
**cephalosporin**
**cephalothin**
**cerebral**
> c. angiography
> c. beriberi
> c. blood flow (CBF)
> c. disorder
> c. edema
> c. embolus
> c. event
> c. infarction
> c. ischemia
> c. perfusion
> c. thrombosis

**cerebritis**
**cerebrovascular**
> c. accident (CVA)
> c. disease
> c. event
> c. insufficiency
> c. thrombosis

**cerebrum**

**cervical**
- c. aortic arch
- c. aortic knuckle
- c. disk
- c. radiculitis
- c. rib syndrome
- c. spine deformity
- c. venous hum

**cervicalis**
- ansa c.

**CF lead**

**Chagas' disease**

**chagoma**

**chain**
- imaging c.

**chamber**
- c. rupture
- c. stiffness

**change**
- STT c.'s

**channel**
- calcium c.
- fast c.
- lymphatic c.
- membrane c.
- receptor-operated calcium c.
- slow c.
- sodium c.
- voltage-dependent calcium c.

**chaotic tachycardia**

**Charcot-Marie-Tooth disease**

**Charcot-Weiss-Baker syndrome**

**Chardack pacemaker**

**CHARGE**
- coloboma, heart disease, atresia choanae, retarded growth, genital hypoplasia, ear anomalies
- CHARGE association syndrome

**charge time**

*[handwritten: CHADS VASC score]*

**Charnley**
- C. drain tube
- C. suction drain

**CHD**
- coronary heart disease

*chelonei*
- *Mycobacterium c.*

**chemical exposure**

**chemodectoma**

**chemoreceptor reflex**

**chemotherapy**

**chemotoxin**

**chenodeoxycholic acid**

**chest**
- c. compression
- foveated c.
- c. leads
- c. pain
- pigeon c.
- c. roentgenogram
- c. roentgenography
- shield c.
- c. wall
- c. x-ray

**Cheyne-Stokes respiration**

**CHF**
- congestive heart failure

**Chiari network**

**chicken fat clot**

*Chlamydia*
- *C. psittaci*
- *C. trachomatis*

**chloride**
- ammonium c.
- Anectine c.
- bethanechol c.
- calcium c.
- edrophonium c.
- c. ion
- polyvinyl c. (PVC)
- potassium c.
- succinylcholine c.
- tubocurarine c.
- xenon c. (XeCl)

chloroquine
chlorothiazide
chlorpromazine
chlortetracycline sensitivity
chlorthalidone
cholecystitis
cholelithiasis
cholera vaccine reaction
cholesterol
    c. embolism
    c. embolization
    c. ester
    c. ester storage disease
    c. pericarditis
cholestyramine
cholinergic receptor
chordae
    c. tendineae
    c. tendineae rupture
chorda tendineae
chordoplasty
chorea
    amyotrophic c.
    c. cordis
    c. gravidarum
    Huntington's c.
    Sydenham's c.
chorionic villus sampling
chromaffin cell tumor
chromic catgut suture
*Chromobacterium*
*Chromosporinum*
chronic
    c. angina
    c. aortic stenosis
    c. constrictive
      pericarditis
    c. hemolytic anemia
    c. hypertensive disease
    c. obstructive pulmonary
      disease (COPD)
    c. renal failure
    c. shock
    c. stable angina

Chronocor pacemaker
chronologic age (CA)
Chronos 04 pacemaker
chronotropic response
chronotropism
    negative c.
    positive c.
Church cardiovascular scissors
Churchill
    C. cardiac suction
      cannula
    C. sucker
Churg-Strauss syndrome
chylomicron
    c. remnant
    c. remnant receptor
chylomicronemia
chylopericarditis
chylopericardium
chylous pericardial effusion
CI
    cardiac index
CI-976
CI-981
cilazapril
cimetidine
cinchonism
cine
    c. camera
    c. computed tomography
    c. pulse system
cineangiocardiography
    radionuclide c.
cineangiogram
cineangiography
    conventional c.
cinecamera
cinefilm
cinefluorography
cinnarizine
Cin-Quin
ciprostene
circadian rhythm

**circulation**
    collateral c.
    compensatory c.
    coronary c.
    coronary collateral c.
    extracorporeal c.
    fetal c.
    left dominant
      coronary c.
    peripheral c.
    persistent fetal c.
    pulmonary c.
    systemic c.
    c. time

**circulatory**
    c. arrest
    c. collapse
    c. congestion
    c. failure
    c. support system
    c. system

**circumferential**
    c. fiber shortening
    c. shortening

**circumflex (CX)**
    c. aortic arch
    c. artery

**circus**
    c. movement tachycardia

**cirrhosis**
    cardiac c.
    congestive c.
    c. of liver
    stasis c.

**cirsoid aneurysm**

**cisternae**
    subsarcolemma c.
    terminal c.

**citrate**
    sufentanil c.

**citric acid cycle**

***Citrobacter***

**CK**
    creatine kinase

**CK-MB**
    myocardial muscle creatine
      kinase isozyme

**clamp**
    Allis c.
    aortic c.
    aortic aneurysm c.
    Beck miniature aortic c.
    bulldog c.
    Bunnell-Howard
      arthrodesis c.
    Calman carotid c.
    Calman ring c.
    cardiovascular c.
    Cooley c.
    Cooley-Beck vessel c.
    Cooley-Derra c.
    Cooley-Satinsky c.
    Cooley vena cava c.
    Crafoord coarctation c.
    Crile c.
    DeBakey c.
    DeBakey-Bahnson c.
    DeBakey-Bainbridge c.
    DeBakey-Beck c.
    DeBakey-Derra
      anastomosis c.
    DeBakey-Harken c.
    DeBakey-Harken
      auricle c.
    DeBakey-Howard c.
    DeBakey-Howard aortic
      aneurysmal c.
    DeBakey-Kay aortic c.
    DeBakey-McQuigg-Mixter
      bronchial c.
    DeBakey-Satinsky vena
      caval c.
    DeBakey-Semb c.
    DeBakey-Semb ligature-
      carrier c.
    Derra c.
    Derra aortic c.
    Derra vena caval c.

DeWeese vena cava c.
Halsted c.
Hartmann c.
Hopkins aortic c.
Hufnagel aortic c.
Hufnagel ascending
 aortic c.
Hunter-Satinsky c.
Jacobson
 microbulldog c.
Jacobson modified
 vessel c.
Jacobson-Potts c.
Javid bypass c.
Javid carotid artery c.
Javid carotid artery
 bypass c.
Kantrowitz thoracic c.
Kelly c.
Lambert-Kay c.
microvascular c.
mosquito c.
Müller vena caval c.
myocardial c.
Pilling
 microanastomosis c.
Rochester-Kocher c.
Rochester-Péan c.
Rumel c.
Sarnoff aortic c.
Satinsky c.
Schumacher aorta c.
Subramanian c.
VascuClamp minibulldog
 vessel c.
VascuClamp vascular c.
vascular c.
vessel c.

**clamshell device**
**Clark**
C. expanding mesh
 catheter
C. helix catheter

C. rotating cutter
 catheter
**classification**
Canadian Cardiovascular
 Society c.
DeBakey c.
functional c.
Killip c.
New York Heart
 Association c.
**claudication**
intermittent c.
**clearance**
airway c.
drug c.
gas c.
c. technique
**cleavage**
abnormal c. of cardiac
 valve
**cleft mitral valve**
**clenched fist sign**
**click**
ejection c.
mitral c.
c. murmur syndrome
systolic c.
**Clinoril**
**clip**
Autostat ligating and
 hemostatic c.'s
Horizon surgical ligating
 and marking c.
ligation c.
micro bulldog c.
Miles vena cava c.
Moretz c.
partial occlusion inferior
 vena cava c.
vascular c.
vena cava c.
**CL lead**
**clofibrate**

**clonidine**
  c. hydrochloride
**clopidogrel**
**closed-chest cardiac massage**
**closing snap**
**clostridial myocarditis**
*Clostridium perfringens*
**closure**
  double umbrella c.
  King ASD umbrella c.
  nonoperative c.
  c. pressure
  primary c.
  transcatheter c.
  umbrella c.
**clot**
  agony c.
  antemortem c.
  blood c.
  chicken fat c.
  currant jelly c.
  laminated c.
  passive c.
  postmortem c.
**clotting**
  c. abnormality
  c. disorder
**clubbing**
**coagulation**
  disseminated
    intravascular c. (DIC)
  c. factor
  c. forceps
  c. necrosis
  c. protein
  c. time
**coagulative myocytolysis**
**coarctation**
  c. of aorta
  aortic c.
  juxtaductal c.
  native c.

  percutaneous balloon
    angioplasty of c.
  c. of pulmonary artery
  reversed c.
**coating**
  Teflon c.
**coaxial pressure**
**cobalt cardiomyopathy**
**Cobe**
  C. cardiotomy reservoir
  C. small vessel cannula
**cocaine abuse**
**cocci**
*Coccidioides*
**coccidioidomycosis**
**coccus, pl. cocci**
**Cockayne's syndrome**
**codeine**
**coefficient**
  damping c.
**coenzyme A**
**coenzyme Q**
**coenzyme Q10**
**coeur en sabot**
**coexistent pathology**
**Cogan's syndrome**
**coil**
  c. embolization
  Gianturco c.
**coincidence detection**
**cold**
  c. blood cardioplegia
  c. exposure
  c. ischemic arrest
  c. pressor test
  c. pressor testing
  c. pressor testing
    maneuver
**Cole-Cecil murmur**
**Colestid**
**colestipol**

*coli*
  Escherichia c.
colic
  biliary c.
colitis
  ulcerative c.
collagen vascular disease
collapse
  cardiovascular c.
  circulatory c.
  hemodynamic c.
  right ventricular
    diastolic c.
collapsing pulse
collar
  locking c.
  c. of Stokes
collateral
  aortopulmonary c.
  bronchial c.
  c. circulation
  c. hyperemia
  systemic c.
  venous c.
  c. vessel
collecting duct
collection
  expired air c.
collimation
collimator
colloid osmotic pressure
coloboma, heart disease,
  atresia choanae, retarded
  growth, genital hypoplasia,
  ear anomalies (CHARGE)
colon
  angiodysplasia of c.
  marginal artery of c.
colonic ischemia
color
  c. Doppler
  c. flow Doppler
color-coded flow mapping

column
  plasma exchange c.
coma
combination beat
combined heart catheterization
commissural fusion
commissurotomy
  mitral c.
  mitral balloon c.
committed mode pacemaker
common carotid artery
community-acquired infection
Compactin
compensated shock
compensation
  depth c.
  electronic distance c.
  workers' c.
compensatory
  c. circulation
  c. hypertrophy of heart
  c. pause
competence
  cardiac c.
complement-fixation test
complement system
complete
  c. atrioventricular
    dissociation
  c. A-V block
  c. A-V dissociation
  c. blood count (CBC)
  c. heart block
  c. pacemaker patient
    testing system (CPTS)
  c. transposition of great
    arteries
completed
  c. myocardial infarction
complex
  aberrant c.
  c. angioplasty
  anomalous c.
  atrial c.

**complex** *(continued)*
    atrial premature c.'s
      (APC)
    auricular c.
    diphasic c.
    Eisenmenger's c.
    electrocardiographic c.
    electrocardiographic
      wave c. (QRS complex)
    equiphasic c.
    isodiphasic c.
    junctional c.
    Lutembacher's c.
    monophasic c.
    multiform premature
      ventricular c.
    plasminogen-
      streptokinase c.
    pleomorphic premature
      ventricular c.
    polymorphic premature
      ventricular c.
    premature atrial c.
    premature
      atrioventricular
      junctional c.
    premature ventricular c.
    prothrombinase c.
    QRS c.
      electrocardiographic
      wave complex
    R-on-T premature
      ventricular c.
    Steidele's c.
    streptokinase-
      plasminogen c.
    transposition c.
    VATER c.
    ventricular c.
**compliance**
    c. of heart
    left ventricular
      chamber c.

    left ventricular
      muscle c.
    patient c.
**complicated myocardial
infarction**
**complication**
    catheterization c.'s
    c. rate
**component**
    elastic c.
**compound**
    antimony c.
    Hurler-Scheie c.
**compression**
    cardiac c.
    chest c.
    intermittent
      pneumatic c.
    c. thrombosis
**Compton**
    C. effect
    C. scatter
**computed**
    c. tomography (CT)
    c. tomography scanner
**computer**
    digital c.
**Comtesse medical support
stockings**
**conal septum**
**concealed**
    c. bypass tract
    c. conduction
**concentric left ventricular
hypertrophy**
**concept**
    leading circle c.
    solid angle c.
**concordance**
    atrioventricular c.
    ventriculoarterial c.
**concordant**
    c. alternans
    c. alternation

concretio cordis
concussion
>myocardial c.
condition
>preexisting c.
conditioning
conductance catheter
conduction
>aberrant c.
>aberrant ventricular c.
>accelerated c.
>antegrade c.
>anterograde c.
>atrioventricular c., A-V c.
>c. block
>cardiac c.
>concealed c.
>decremental c.
>c. defect
>c. delay
>delayed c.
>c. disturbance
>forward c.
>impulse c.
>interatrial c.
>internodal c.
>intra-atrial c.
>intraventricular c.
>c. pathway
>Purkinje c.
>retrograde c.
>supernormal c.
>supranormal c.
>c. system
>c. time
>ventricular c.
>ventriculoatrial c., V-A c.
conductive coupling
configuration
>atrial sensing c.
>spike-and-dome c.
>ventricular sensing c.

congenita
>myotonia c.
congenital
>c. adrenal hyperplasia
>c. aortic aneurysm
>c. aortic stenosis
>c. heart block
>c. heart disease
>c. interrupted aortic arch
>c. mitral stenosis
>c. single atrium
congenitally absent pericardium
congested
congestion
>active c.
>circulatory c.
>functional c.
>hypostatic c.
>passive c.
>physiologic c.
>venous c.
congestive
>c. cardiomyopathy
>c. cirrhosis
>c. heart failure (CHF)
conjunctiva
connection
>anomalous pulmonary venous c.
>pulmonary venous c.
>systemic-to-pulmonary c.
>total anomalous pulmonary venous c.
>univentricular atrioventricular c.
connective tissue
connector
>Biotronik lead c.
>cordis c.
>Luer-Lok c.
>Medtronic c.
>unipolar c.

Conn's syndrome
conoventricular fold and groove
Conradi-Hünermann syndrome
Conradi's line
Conray
consanguinity
consciousness
    loss of c.
consent
    informed c.
constant
    c. coupling
    empiric c.
    gas c. (R)
    Gorlin c.
    Hodgkin-Huxley c.
constriction
    occult pericardial c.
constrictive
    c. endocarditis
    c. heart disease
    c. pericarditis
    c. physiology
consumption
    myocardial oxygen c.
    oxygen c.
content
    harmonic c.
    oxygen c.
continuity equation
continuous
    c. heart murmur
    c. murmur
    c. positive airway pressure (CPAP)
continuous-wave
    c.-w. Doppler
    c.-w. Doppler echocardiography
    c.-w. Doppler ultrasound
    c.-w. laser ablation

contour
    c. of heart
    ventricular c.
contraceptive
    c. agent
    oral c.
contracta
    vena c.
contractile
    c. element
    c. function
    c. protein
contractility
    myocardial c.
    ventricular c.
contraction
    anodal closure c.
    anodal opening c.
    atrial premature c.
    automatic c.
    automatic ventricular c.
    c. band
    c. band necrosis
    cardiac c.
    escaped c.
    escaped ventricular c.
    Gowers' c.
    isometric c.
    isotonic c.
    nodal premature c.
    c. pattern
    premature c.
    premature atrial c. (PAC)
    premature ventricular c. (PVC)
    supraventricular premature c.
    ventricular premature c.
contracture
    ischemic c. of left ventricle
contraindication

**contrast**
    c. agent
    c. allergic patient
    c. echocardiography
    c. material
    c. medium
    c. medium delivery
    negative c.
    Optiray c.
    c. ratio
    c. ventriculography
**control**
    axial c.
    damping c.
    gain c.
    quality c.
    reject c.
    time-varied gain c.
      (TGC)
    torque c.
    c. wire
**contusion**
    cardiac c.
    myocardial c.
**conus**
    c. arteriosus
    c. cordis
    c. ligament
**convalescence**
**conventional cineangiography**
**conversion**
    analog-to-digital c.
    pressure c.
**converter**
    scan c.
**converting enzyme inhibitor**
**convulsion**
**Cook**
    C. flexible biopsy
      forceps
    C. intracoronary stent
**Cooley**
    C. clamp
    C. dilator

    C. retractor
    C. vena cava clamp
**Cooley's anemia**
**Cooley-Beck vessel clamp**
**Cooley-Derra clamp**
**Cooley-Satinsky clamp**
**cooling**
    cardioplegia c.
    core c.
**Coombs murmur**
**coordinate system**
**COPD**
    chronic obstructive
    pulmonary disease
**copper (CU)**
**copper-62 ($^{62}$CU)**
**cor**, gen. **cordis**
    c. adiposum
    c. biloculare
    c. bovinum
    c. dextrum
    c. en cuirasse
    c. mobile
    c. pendulum
    c. pulmonale
    c. sinistrum
    c. taurinum
    c. triatriatum
    c. triloculare, c.
      triloculare biatriatum, c.
      triloculare biventriculare
**Coratomic**
    C. implantable pulse
      generator
    C. pacemaker
**Cordarone**
**Cordis**
    C. bioptome
    C. catheter
    C. pacemaker
**cordis**
    accretio c.
    angina c.
    annuli fibrosi c.

**cordis** *(continued)*
    apex c.
    bulbus c.
    concretio c.
    c. connector
    conus c.
    crena c.
    ectopia c.
    c. leads
    myopathia c.
    paracentesis c.
    c. sheath
    trepidatio c.
    tumultus c.
**cordy pulse**
**core cooling**
**Corgard**
**Cori's disease**
**Corlopam**
**cornae**
    arcus c.
**Cornelia de Lange syndrome**
**coronarism**
**coronaritis**
**Coronary**
    C. Artery Surgery Study
    (CASS)
    C. Primary Prevention
    Trial (CPPT)
**coronary**
    c. aneurysm
    c. angiographic catheter
    c. angiography
    c. angioplasty
    c. arterial reserve
    c. arteriography
    c. arteriosclerosis
    c. artery
    c. artery anomaly
    c. artery atherosclerosis
    c. artery bypass graft
    (CABG)
    c. artery bypass grafting
    surgery

c. artery bypass surgery
c. artery disease (CAD)
c. artery dissection
c. artery ectasia
c. artery fistula
c. artery lesion
c. artery obstruction
c. artery occlusion
c. artery probe
c. artery-right ventricular
  fistula
c. artery spasm
c. artery stenosis
c. artery thrombosis
c. atherectomy
c. atherosclerosis
c. bifurcation
c. blood flow (CBF)
c. blood flow
  measurement
c. bypass
c. bypass graft surgery
c. bypass surgery
café c.
c. care unit (CCU)
c. circulation
c. collateral circulation
c. embolism
c. endarterectomy
c. failure
c. flow reserve
c. flow reserve
  technique
c. heart disease (CHD)
c. insufficiency
c. nodal rhythm
c. occlusion
c. occlusive disease
c. ostial stenosis
c. ostium
c. roadmapping
c. seeking catheter
c. sinus
c. sinus catheterization

c. sinus electrogram
c. sinus rhythm
c. sinus thermodilution
c. spasm
c. steal
c. steal mechanism
c. stenosis
c. sulcus
c. thrombolysis
c. thrombosis
c. vascular reserve
c. vascular resistance
c. vascular turgor
c. vasodilation
c. vasodilator reserve
c. vasomotion
c. vasospasm
c. vein
c. venous pressure
**corrected dextrocardia**
**Corrigan's**
C. disease
C. pulse
*corrodens*
*Eikenella c.*
**corticosteroid**
**cortisol**
**Corvisart's facies**
**Corwin**
*Corynebacterium*
**Corzide**
**Cosmos pacemaker**
**Cosprin**
**cost-benefit analysis**
**cost-effectiveness analysis**
**costochondral syndrome**
**costochondritis**
**costoclavicular rib syndrome**
**costosternal syndrome**
**costovertebral angle (CVA)**
**cosyntropin**
**cotton-wool spot**
**cough syncope**
**Coumadin**

**coumadinization**
**coumarin**
**Coumel's tachycardia**
**counseling**
genetic c.
retrospective genetic c.
**count**
blood c.
complete blood c. (CBC)
end-diastolic c.
end-systolic c.
first shock c.
c. rate
second through fifth shock c.
total patient shock c.
white blood cell c.
**counterpulsation**
intra-arterial c.
**countershock**
electrical c.
**count-rate linearity**
**coupled**
c. beat
c. pulse
c. rhythm
**couplets**
**coupling**
arterial c.
conductive c.
constant c.
electromechanical c.
excitation-contraction c.
fixed c.
c. interval
variable c.
ventriculoarterial c.
**Cournand**
C. catheter
C. needle
C. quadpolar catheter
**Cournand's dip**
*Coxiella burnetii*

**Cox proportional hazard model**
**Coxsackievirus**
**Coxsackievirus A**
**Coxsackievirus B**
**coxsackievirus myocarditis**
**CPAP**
  continuous positive airway pressure
**CPB**
  cardiopulmonary bypass
**CPI PRX implantable cardioverter-defibrillator**
**CPK**
  creatine phosphokinase
**CPPT**
  Coronary Primary Prevention Trial
**CPR**
  cardiopulmonary resuscitation
**CPTS**
  complete pacemaker patient testing system
**Crafoord coarctation clamp**
**Crampton test**
**cranial arteritis**
**craniocardiac reflex**
**crassamentum**
**Crawford suture ring**
**cream**
  Synapse electrocardiographic c.
**creatine**
  c. kinase (CK)
  c. phosphokinase (CPK)
**creatinine**
**Creech technique**
**creeping thrombosis**
**crena**, pl. **crenae**
  c. cordis
**crescendo**
  c. angina
  c. murmur

**crescendo-decrescendo murmur**
**Cribier-Letac**
  C.-L. aortic valvuloplasty balloon
  C.-L. balloon
  C.-L. catheter
**cri du chat syndrome**
**Crile**
  C. clamp
  C. tip occluder
**crisis**
  hypertensive c.
**Crisp's aneurysm**
**crisscross**
  c. atrioventricular valve
  c. heart
  c. heart malposition
**crista**
  c. supraventricularis
  c. terminalis
**criteria**
  Dallas c.
  exclusion c.
  Heath-Edwards c.
  Jones c.
  voltage c.
**critical**
  c. care
  c. rate
**Criticare**
  C. ETCO2 multigas analyzer
  C. ETCO2/SpO2 monitor
  C. pulse oximeter
**Critikon**
  C. balloon temporary pacing catheter
  C. balloon wedge pressure catheter
**CR lead**
**cromolyn sodium**
**crossclamp**
  aortic c.

crossed embolism
cross-linkage theory
cross-reactive antibody
cross-sectional
    echocardiography
*Crotalus*
cruces
cruces
crus, pl. crura
    c. dextrum fasciculi
        atrioventricularis
    c. sinistrum fasciculi
        atrioventricularis
Cruveilhier-Baumgarten
    C.-B. murmur
    C.-B. sign
crux, pl. cruces
    c. of heart
*cruzi*
    *Trypanosoma c.*
cryoablation
cryoglobulinemia
cryoprecipitate
cryptococcosis
*Cryptococcus neoformans*
crystalloid fluid
CT
    computed tomography
CU
    copper
$^{62}$CU
    copper-62
cuff
    blood pressure c.
cuffing
    peribronchial c.
cuirasse
    cor en c.
culture-negative endocarditis
cuprophane membrane
curare
currant jelly clot
current
    bioelectric c.

diastolic c.
K c.
pump c.
systolic c.
transient inward c.
curve
    actuarial survival c.
    Frank-Starling c.
    function c.
    hemoglobin-oxygen
        dissociation c.
    intracardiac pressure c.
    Kaplan Meier
        survival c.
    left ventricular pressure-
        volume c.
    length-active tension c.
    pressure-natriuresis c.
    pressure-volume c.
    pulse c.
    Starling c.
    time-activity c.
    venous return c.
    venovenous dye
        dilution c.
    ventricular function c.
    volume-time c.
curved j-exchange wire
cushingoid
    c. facies
Cushing pressure response
Cushing's syndrome
cusp eversion
cutdown
    arterial c.
    brachial artery c.
    c. technique
    venous c.
cutis
    c. laxa
    c. laxa syndrome
CVA
    cerebrovascular accident
    costovertebral angle

**CVP**
    central venous pressure
*c* wave
**CX**
    circumflex
**cyanochroic, cyanochrous**
**cyanosed**
**cyanose tardive**
**cyanosis**
    tardive c.
**cyanotic**
    c. asphyxia
    c. atrophy of liver
    c. defect
    c. heart defect
**Cyberlith pacemaker**
**cyclase**
    adenylate c.
**cycle**
    cardiac c.
    citric acid c.
    forced c.
    restored c.
    returning c.
    sound wave c.
    Wenckebach c.

**cycle-length window**
**cyclic**
    c. adenosine
        monophosphate (cAMP)
    c. respiration
**cyclooxygenase inhibitor**
**cyclopenthiazide**
**cyclophosphamide**
**cyclopropane**
**cyclosporine**
**cyclothiazide**
**Cynosar catheter**
**cyst**
    echinococcal c.
    hydatid c.
    pericardial c.
    renal c.
**cysteine**
**cystic**
    c. fibrosis
    c. medial necrosis
**cysticercosis**
**cytomegalic inclusion disease**
**cytomegalovirus**
**cytosine arabinoside (CA)**

*D-dimer test*

DaCosta's syndrome
Dacron
- D. catheter
- D. graft
- D. intracardiac patch
- D. patch
- D. pledget

DAH
- disordered action of heart

Dallas criteria
damping
- d. coefficient
- d. control

dance
- hilar d.
- St. Vitus d.

dantrolene sodium
Datascope balloon
Datex ETCO2 multigas analyzer
Davies' disease
dazoxiben
DBP
- diastolic blood pressure

DCA
- directional coronary atherectomy

DDAVP
- desmopressin acetate

DDD pacing
DDDR pacing
DDI pacing
dead time
deaminase
- adenosine d.

D to E amplitude
death
- brain d.
- cardiac d.
- late d.
- sudden d.

sudden cardiac d.
voodoo d.

DeBakey
- D. clamp
- D. classification
- D. tissue forceps

DeBakey-Bahnson clamp
DeBakey-Bainbridge clamp
DeBakey-Beck clamp
DeBakey-Derra anastomosis clamp
DeBakey-Harken
- D.-H. auricle clamp
- D.-H. clamp

DeBakey-Howard
- D.-H. aortic aneurysmal clamp
- D.-H. clamp

DeBakey-Kay aortic clamp
DeBakey-McQuigg-Mixter bronchial clamp
DeBakey-Satinsky vena caval clamp
DeBakey-Semb
- D.-S. clamp
- D.-S. ligature-carrier clamp

debility
- reversible ischemic neurologic d. (RIND)

debris
- calcific d.
- valve d.

debrisoquine sulfate
decay
- pressure d.

deceleration
- early d.
- late d.
- variable d.

2-D echocardiography
Decholin

declamping shock
decompensated shock
decompensation
decompression sickness
deconditioning
decrement
decremental conduction
decrescendo murmur
decubitus ulcer
deductive echocardiography
deep hypothermia circulatory
  arrest (DHCA)
de-epicardialization
deep venous thrombosis
  (DVT)
defecation syncope
defect
    aorticopulmonary d.
    aortic septal d.,
      aorticopulmonary
      septal d.
    atrial septal d. (ASD)
    atrioseptal d.
    atrioventricular canal d.
    atrioventricular septal d.
    conduction d.
    cyanotic d.
    cyanotic heart d.
    endocardial cushion d.
    iatrogenic atrial
      septal d.
    ostium primum d.
    ostium secundum d.
    panconduction d.
    perfusion d.
    perimembranous
      ventricular septal d.
    primum atrial septal d.
    septal d.
    sinus venosus d.
    Swiss cheese d.
    ventricular septal d.
      (VSD)
defibrillation

defibrillator
    automatic implantable d.
    automatic intracardiac d.
    cardioverter-d.
    external d.
    Ventak d.
deficiency
    acid maltase d.
    dopamine beta-
      hydroxylase d.
    galactosidase d.
    glucosidase d.
    hexosaminidase d.
    homogentisic acid
      oxidase d.
    hydroxylase d.
    17-hydroxylase d.
    maltase d.
    protein-calorie d.
    selenium d.
    thiamine d.
    vasopressor d.
deficit
    pulse d.
definitive surgery
deflated profile
deflection
    intrinsic d.
    intrinsicoid d.
deformity
    cervical spine d.
    gooseneck d.
    joint d.
    parachute d.
degeneration
    fibrinoid d.
    Mönckeberg's d.
    mucoid medial d.
    myxomatous d.
    Quain's d.
    spinocerebellar d.
degenerative
deglutition syncope
Degos' disease

Dehio's test
dehiscence
dehydroemetine
dehydrogenase
    glucose-6-phosphate d.
    lactate d.
    lactic acid d.
    pyruvate d.
de Lange's syndrome
delay
    conduction d.
    intraventricular
     conduction d.
delayed
    d. afterdepolarization
    d. conduction
Delbet's sign
delirium cordis
delivery
    contrast medium d.
    d. wire
delta wave
demand
    myocardial oxygen d.
    d. pacemaker
    d. pulse generator
De Martel scissors
Demerol
de Musset's sign
denial
de novo lesion
density
    hydrogen d.
    proton d.
    spin d.
density-exposure relationship
  of film
dental procedure
2-deoxyglucose
deoxyribonuclease (DNase)
deoxyribonucleic acid (DNA)
dependence
    use d.
dependent beat

depolarization
    atrial premature d.'s
    diastolic d.
    myocardial d.
    rapid d.
    transient d.
Deponit
deposition
    calcium oxalate d.
depression
    aldosterone d.
    myocardial d.
    postdrive d.
depressor reflex
Depthalon
depth compensation
derivative
    hematoporphyrin d.
    (HPD)
dermatan sulfate
*dermatitidis*
    *Blastomyces d.*
dermatitis, pl. dermatitides
    exfoliative d.
dermatomyositis
Derra
    D. aortic clamp
    D. clamp
    D. vena caval clamp
DES
    diethylstilbestrol
descending aorta
descent
    x d.
    y d.
Deseret flow-directed
  thermodilution catheter
desferrioxamine
Desilets-Hoffman sheath
desipramine hydrochloride
deslanoside
D to E slope
desmopressin acetate
  (DDAVP)

**Desyrel**
**detection**
    automated edge d.
    coincidence d.
    edge d.
    manual edge d.
    shunt d.
    single-photon d.
**detective quantum efficiency**
**detector**
    VEST left ventricular
    function d.
**determination**
    metabolic parameter d.
**DeVega annuloplasty**
**developer**
    film d.
**deviation**
    abnormal left axis d.
    (ALAD)
    abnormal right axis d.
    (ARAD)
    axis d.
    left axis d. (LAD)
    right axis d. (RAD)
**device**
    Adams-DeWeese d.
    atrial septal defect
    single disk closure d.
    BIVAD centrifugal left
    and right d.
    Cath-Lok catheter
    locking d.
    clamshell d.
    Elecath circulatory
    support d.
    intra-aortic balloon d.
    intracaval d.
    left ventricular assist d.
    (LVAD)
    locking d.
    right ventricular
    assist d. (RVAD)
    rotary atherectomy d.

    snare d.
    transvenous d.
    ventricular assist d.
    (VAD)
**DeWeese vena cava clamp**
**dexamethasone suppression**
    **test**
**dexedrine**
**dexiocardia**
**dexter**
**dextran**
    high-molecular-weight d.
**dextran 70**
**dextroamphetamine toxicity**
**dextrocardia, dexiocardia**
    corrected d.
    false d.
    isolated d.
    d. malposition
    mirror-image d.
    secondary d.
    type 1 d.
    type 2 d.
    type 3 d.
    type 4 d.
    d. with situs inversus
**dextrocardiogram**
**dextrogastria**
**dextrogram**
**dextroisomerism**
**dextroposition**
    d. of heart
**dextrothyroxine**
**dextrotransposition**
**dextroversion**
    d. of heart
**dextrum**
    cor d.
**DFP**
    diastolic filling pressure
**d gate**
**DHCA**
    deep hypothermia
    circulatory arrest

**diabetic**
    d. cardiomyopathy
    d. diet
    d. nephropathy
    d. ulcer
**diabeticorum**
    necrobiosis d.
    necrobiosis lipoidica d.
**diacylglycerol**
    d. lipase
**diagnosis**
    differential d.
    etiologic d.
    prenatal d.
**diagnosis-related group (DRG)**
**diagnostic testing**
**diagonal artery**
**diagram**
    ladder d.
    pressure-volume d.
**dialysis**
    peritoneal d.
    renal d.
**diameter**
    anteroposterior
     thoracic d.
    internal d.
    stretched d.
    total end-diastolic d.
     (TEDD)
    total end-systolic d.
     (TESD)
**diamond-shaped murmur**
**Diamox**
**diaphragm**
    d. transducer
**diaphragmatic**
    d. flutter
    d. myocardial infarction
**Diaqua**
**diastasis**
**diastatic**
**diastole**
    cardiac d.

**diastolic**
    d. afterpotential
    d. blood pressure (DBP)
    d. closing velocity
    d. current
    d. current of injury
    d. depolarization
    d. doming
    d. dysfunction
    d. filling
    d. filling period
    d. filling pressure (DFP)
    d. fluttering
    d. fluttering aortic valve
    d. function
    d. heart disease
    d. heart failure
    d. hump
    d. hypertension
    d. motion
    d. murmur
    d. overload
    d. pressure
    d. pressure-time index
     (DPTI)
    d. pressure-volume
     relation
    d. relaxation
    d. reserve
    d. rumble
    d. shock
    d. stiffness
    d. suction
    d. thrill
    d. upstroke
**diathermy**
**diatrizoate**
    sodium meglumine d.
**diazepam**
**diazotrate**
**diazoxide**
**Dibenzyline**

**DIC**
    disseminated intravascular
    coagulation
**dichloroisoprenaline**
**dichloroisoproterenol**
**dicrotic**
    d. notch
    d. pulse
    d. wave
**dicrotism**
**Dicumarol**
**dielectrography**
**diet**
    American Heart
      Association d.
    diabetic d.
    high fiber d.
    low fat d.
    low salt d.
    low sodium d.
    renal d.
**dietary**
    d. fat
    d. salt
    d. sodium
**diethylstilbestrol (DES)**
**difference**
    arteriovenous oxygen d.
**differential**
    d. blood pressure
    d. diagnosis
**differentiation**
    echocardiographic d.
**diffuse intimal thickening**
**diffusing capacity**
**diffusum**
    angiokeratoma
      corporis d.
**digammacarboxy-glutamic acid**
**DiGeorge syndrome**
**digestive system vascular
  disease**
**digital**
    d. angiography

d. averaging
d. computer
d. echocardiography
d. fluoroscopic unit
d. smoothing
d. subtraction
d. subtraction
  angiography (DSA)
d. subtraction
  arteriography
d. subtraction technique
**digitalis**
    d. glycoside
    d. intoxication
    d. sensitivity
**digitalis-specific antibody**
**digitalization**
**digitization**
**digitoxin**
**digoxin**
**dihydralazine**
**dihydroergotamine**
**Dilacor**
**Dilantin**
**dilatancy**
**dilated cardiomyopathy**
**dilation, dilatation**
    balloon d.
    bootstrap d.
    finger d.
    idiopathic d.
    reactive d.
    serial d.
    d. thrombosis
    ventricular d.
**dilator**
    argon vessel d.
    Cooley d.
    Encapsulon vessel d.
    Garrett d.
    Mullins d.
    Scanlan vessel d.
    d. and sheath technique

Tubbs d.
vessel d.
**dilator-sheath system**
**dilevalol**
**diltiazem**
d. hydrochloride
**dimension**
end-diastolic d.
end-systolic d.
left atrial d.
left ventricular
internal d.
right ventricular d.
**dimethyl hydrazine**
**dinitrate**
isosorbide d.
**dinucleotide**
nicotinamide adenine d.
(NAD)
**dioxide**
carbon d.
**dip**
Cournand's d.
d. phenomenon
type I d.
type II d.
**diphasic complex**
**diphenhydramine**
**diphenylhydantoin**
**diphosphate**
adenosine d. (ADP)
**5'-diphosphate**
**2,3-diphosphoglycerate**
**diphtheria**
**diplocardia**
**dipole theory**
**dipyridamole**
**dipyridamole-thallium imaging**
**direct**
d. cardiac puncture
d. embolism
d. insertion technique
d. lead
**direct-current cardioversion**

**directional coronary**
**atherectomy (DCA)**
**Dirythmin**
**Dirythmin SA**
**disability**
cardiovascular d.
**disc**
**disc-cage valve**
**discordance**
atrioventricular d.
ventriculoarterial d.
**discordant**
d. alternans
d. alternation
**discrete**
d. subaortic stenosis
d. subvalvular aortic
stenosis
**disease**
Adams-Stokes d.
Addison's d.
amyloid heart d.
aortic aneurysmal d.
aortic
thromboembolic d.
aortic valve d.
aortoiliac occlusive d.
atherosclerotic d.
atherosclerotic aortic d.
Ayerza's d.
Becker's d.
Behçet's d.
biliary d.
Binswanger's d.
Bouillaud's d.
Bright's d.
Buerger's d.
carcinoid heart d.
carcinoid valve d.
cerebrovascular d.
Chagas' d.
Charcot-Marie-Tooth d.
cholesterol ester
storage d.

**disease** *(continued)*
    chronic hypertensive d.
    chronic obstructive
      pulmonary d. (COPD)
    collagen vascular d.
    congenital heart d.
    constrictive heart d.
    Cori's d.
    coronary artery d.
      (CAD)
    coronary heart d.
      (CHD)
    coronary occlusive d.
    Corrigan's d.
    cytomegalic inclusion d.
    Davies' d.
    Degos' d.
    diastolic heart d.
    digestive system
      vascular d.
    Duroziez' d.
    Ebstein's d.
    Eisenmenger's d.
    electrical d.
    Emery-Dreifuss d.
    endomyocardial d.
    end-stage renal d.
    Erdheim d.
    Fabry's d.
    fibroplastic d.
    Friedreich's d.
    Gairdner's d.
    gallbladder d.
    Gaucher's d.
    glycogen storage d.
    gonadal d.
    Graves d.
    Hamman's d.
    Hand-Schüller-
      Christian d.
    heart d.
    hematologic d.
    hepatic d.
    Hodgkin's d.

    Hodgson's d.
    humeroperoneal
      neuromuscular d.
    hypertensive pulmonary
      vascular d.
    iron storage d.
    ischemic heart d.
    Kawasaki's d.
    Keshan d.
    Kugelberg-Welander d.
    large-vessel d.
    left main coronary
      artery d.
    Legionnaires' d.
    Lenègre's d.
    Lev's d.
    Little's d.
    Löffler's d.
    luetic d.
    Lyme d.
    McArdle's d.
    metastatic d.
    Mondor's d.
    Monge's d.
    Morgagni's d.
    moyamoya d.
    multivalvular d.
    multivessel d.
    myocardial d.
    neoplastic d.
    neuromuscular d.
    Niemann-Pick d.
    obstructive lung d.
    occlusive d.
    Paget's d.
    pericardial d.
    peripheral
      atherosclerotic d.
    peripheral vascular d.
    Plummer's d.
    polycystic kidney d.
    polysaccharide storage d.
    Pompe's d.
    pulmonary d.

pulmonary valve d.
pulmonary vascular d.
pulmonary vascular
  obstructive d.
pulmonary veno-
  occlusive d.
pulseless d.
Raynaud's d.
Refsum's d.
Reiter's d.
renal d.
renal artery d.
renal parenchymal d.
Rendu-Osler-Weber d.
restrictive heart d.
restrictive lung d.
rheumatic heart d.
Roger's d.
Rougnon-Heberden d.
Roussy-Lévy d.
Sandhoff's d.
Shoshin d.
sickle cell d.
single-vessel d.
sinus node d.
spirochetal d.
Steinert's d.
Still's d.
Stokes-Adams d.
Takayasu-Ohnishi d.
Takayasu's d.
Tangier d.
Taussig-Bing d.
Tay-Sachs d.
Thomsen's d.
thromboembolic d.
thyrocardiac d.
thyroid d.
thyrotoxic heart d.
traumatic heart d.
tricuspid valve d.
valvular heart d.
Vaquez's d.

vertebrobasilar
  occlusive d.
vibration d.
von Recklinghausen's d.
von Willebrand's d.
Weber-Christian d.
Weil's d.
Wilkie's d.
Wilson's d.
Winiwarter-Buerger d.
**disintegration rate**
**disk, disc**
  cervical d.
  intervertebral d.
  optic d.
  d. spring
**disopyramide**
**disorder**
  autoimmune d.
  cerebral d.
  clotting d.
  endocrine d.
  genetic d.
  glycosphingolipid d.
  iatrogenic d.
  mendelian d.
  movement d.
  neurological d.
  neuromuscular d.
  neuromyopathic d.
  panic d.
  single-gene d.
**disordered action of heart
  (DAH)**
**dispersing electrode**
**dispersion**
  temporal d.
**displacement**
**Disprin**
**disruption**
  traumatic aortic d.
**dissecting**
  d. aortic aneurysm
  d. hematoma

**dissection**
  d. of aorta
  aortic d.
  arterial d.
  coronary artery d.
**disseminated intravascular coagulation (DIC)**
**dissociation**
  atrial d.
  atrioventricular d., A-V d.
  complete atrioventricular d., complete A-V d.
  electromechanical d.
  incomplete atrioventricular d., incomplete A-V d.
  interference d.
  isorhythmic d.
  longitudinal d.
**dissolution**
**distal**
  d. convoluted tubule
  d. end
**distance**
  half-power d.
**distensibility**
  ventricular d.
**distention**
  jugular venous d. (JVD)
**distortion**
  pincushion d.
**distress**
  respiratory d.
**distribution**
  blood volume d.
  volume of d.
**distributive shock**
**disturbance**
  conduction d.
  rhythm d.
**disulfide**
  carbon d.

**Dittrich's stenosis**
**Diucardin**
**Diulo**
**diuretic**
  cardiac d.
  indirect d.
  loop d.
  osmotic d.
  potassium-sparing d.
  thiazide d.
**Diurexan**
**Diuril**
**diver's syncope**
**diverticula**
**divisional**
  d. block
  d. heart block
**Divistyramine**
**dizziness**
**d loop**
**DNA**
  deoxyribonucleic acid
**DNase**
  deoxyribonuclease
**dobutamine stress echocardiography (DSC)**
**Dobutrex**
**docosahexaenoic acid**
**dolens**
  phlegmasia alba d.
  phlegmasia cerulea d.
**dolichostenomelia**
**dome excursion**
**dome-shaped**
**doming**
  diastolic d.
  systolic d.
  tricuspid valve d.
**domperidone**
L-**dopa**
**dopamine beta-hydroxylase deficiency**
**dopaminergic agent**
**Dopastat**

**dopexamine**
**Doppler**
 D. cardiography
 carotid D.
 D. catheter
 color D.
 color flow D.
 D. continuity equation
 continuous-wave D.
 D. echocardiography
 D. effect
 D. equation
 D. measurement
 D. pressure gradient
 pulsed D.
 pulsed D.
  echocardiography
 D. recording
 D. shift
 D. signal
 D. study
 D. technique
 D. transducer
 D. ultrasonography
 D. ultrasound
 D. velocity probe
**Dorendorf's sign**
**dorsalis pedis pulse**
**dosage regimen**
**dose**
 radiation absorbed d.
  (rad)
**Dotter technique**
**double**
 d. aortic arch
 d. aortic stenosis
 d. disc occluder
 d. product
 d. tachycardia
 d. umbrella
 d. umbrella closure
**double-balloon**
 d.-b. catheter

 d.-b. valvotomy
 d.-b. valvuloplasty
**double-inlet ventricle**
**double-lumen catheter**
**double-outlet**
 d.-o. left ventricle
 d.-o. left ventricle
  malposition
 d.-o. right ventricle
 d.-o. right ventricle
  malposition
**double-shock sound**
**doughnut sign**
**Douglas**
 D. bag
 D. bag method
 D. bag technique
**down-regulation**
**Down's syndrome**
**doxazosin**
 d. mesylate
**doxepin**
 d. hydrochloride
**doxorubicin cardiomyopathy**
**dP/dt**
**dP/dt$_{MAX}$-end-diastolic volume**
**(dP/dt)/P**
**(dP/dt)/P$_D$**
**dP/dt/TP**
**DPTI**
 diastolic pressure-time index
**drain**
 Charnley suction d.
**drainage**
 anomalous pulmonary
  venous d.
 pulmonary venous d.
**Dressler beat**
**Dressler's syndrome**
**DRG**
 diagnosis-related group
**Dr. Gibaud thermal health
 support**
**drift**

**drill-tip catheter**
**droperidol**
**drop heart**
**dropped beat**
**drug**
d. abuse
anthracycline d.
antituberculous d.
d. clearance
pressor d.
sympathomimetic d.
vasoactive d.
**drug-associated pericarditis**
**Drummond**
marginal arteries of D.
**Drummond's sign**
**dry beriberi**
**drying**
film d.
d. film
**DSA**
digital subtraction
angiography
**DSC**
dobutamine stress
echocardiography
**d-TGA**
d-transposition of great
arteries
**d-transposition of great
arteries (d-TGA)**
**dual**
d. chamber pacemaker
d. demand pacemaker
d. echophono-
cardiography
**dual-chamber pacing**
**Du Bois-Reymond's law**
**Duchenne's**
D. dystrophy
D. muscular dystrophy
**Ducor catheter**
**duct**
collecting d.

medullary collecting d.
thoracic d.
**ductus**
d. arteriosus
d. venosus
**Duostat rotating hemostatic
valve**
**Duotrate 30**
**Duotrate 45**
**duplex scanning**
**Duraflow heart valve**
**Duran annuloplasty ring**
**Duraquin**
**duration**
half amplitude pulse d.
pulse d.
**Duromedics prosthesis**
**Duroziez'**
D. disease
D. murmur
D. sign
D. symptom
**duty factor**
**DVI pacing**
**DVT**
deep venous thrombosis
**dwarfism**
aortic d.
**Dyazide**
**dye**
d. dilution method
flash-lamp excited
pulsed d.
indocyanine green d.
d. method
radiocontrast d.
**DynaCirc**
**dynamic**
d. aorta
d. exercise
d. frequency response
d. murmur
d. pressure
d. range

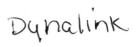

**dynamics**
    fluid d.
    funnel d.
    left ventricular-left atrial
      crossover d.
**Dyrenium**
**dysarteriotony**
**dysautonomia**
    familial d.
**dysbetalipoproteinemia**
**dyscrasia**
    blood d.
**dysfibrinogenemia**
**dysfunction**
    diastolic d.
    intellectual d.
    left ventricular d.
    papillary muscle d.
    sinus node d.
    valvular d.
**dysgenesis**
    gonadal d.
**dyskinesia**
**dyskinesis**
**dysphagia, dysphagy**
**dysplasia**
    arrhythmogenic right
      ventricular d.
    fibromuscular d.
    fibrous d.

    polyostotic fibrous d.
    right ventricular d.
    ventriculoradial d.
**dysplastic**
**dyspnea**
    exertional d.
    functional d.
    inspiratory d.
    nocturnal d.
    paroxysmal nocturnal d.
    (PND)
**dysrhythmia**
    cardiac d.
**dyssynchrony**
**dystrophin**
**dystrophy**
    Becker d.
    Becker-type tardive
      muscular d.
    Duchenne's d.
    Duchenne's muscular d.
    Emery-Dreifuss
      muscular d.
    facioscapulohumeral d.
    Landouzy-Déjérine d.
    limb-girdle muscular d.
    muscular d.
    myotonic d.
    myotonic muscular d.

**Ea**
 effective arterial elastance
**early**
 e. afterdepolarization
 e. deceleration
 e. diastolic murmur
 e. rapid repolarization
 e. systolic murmur
**early-peaking systolic murmur**
**ear oximeter**
**Easprin**
**EBDA**
 effective balloon dilating
 area
**Ebstein's**
 E. anomaly
 E. anomaly of tricuspid
 valve
 E. disease
 E. sign
**eccentricity index**
**eccentric stenosis**
**ecchymotic mask**
**ECG**
 electrocardiogram
**echinococcal cyst**
**echinococcosis**
*Echinococcus*
**echo**
 atrial e.
 e. beat
 e. delay time (TE)
 e. guidance
 motion display e.
 nodus sinuatrialis e.,
 NS e.
 e. ranging
 scattered e.
 e. score
 specular e.
 transcutaneous e.
 transesophageal e.

**echoaortography**
**echocardiographic**
 e. assessment
 e. differentiation
 e. scoring system
 e. transducer
**echocardiography**
 A-mode e.
 B-mode e.
 continuous-wave
 Doppler e.
 contrast e.
 cross-sectional e.
 2-D e.
 deductive e.
 digital e.
 dobutamine stress e.
 (DSC)
 Doppler e.
 esophageal e.
 exercise e.
 interventional e.
 intrauterine e.
 12-lead e.
 mitral valve e.
 M-mode e.
 pulmonary valve e.
 pulsed Doppler e.
 real-time e.
 three-dimensional e.
 transesophageal e. (TEE)
 two-dimensional e.
**echo-Doppler cardiography**
**echogram**
**echophonocardiography**
 dual e.
**echoscope**
**ECHO virus**
**echovirus myocarditis**
**ECLA**
 excimer laser coronary
 angioplasty

**eclampsia**
**ectasia, ectasis**
annuloaortic e.
artery e.
e. cordis
coronary artery e.
**ectocardia**
**ectocardiac, ectocardial**
**ectopia**
e. cordis
e. cordis malposition
e. lentis
**ectopic**
e. atrial tachycardia
e. beat
e. impulse
e. pacemaker
e. rhythm
e. tachycardia
**ectopy**
supraventricular e.
ventricular e.
**ECT pacemaker**
**eddy sounds**
**Edecrin**
**edema**
alveolar e.
angioneurotic e.
cardiac e.
cardiogenic
pulmonary e.
cerebral e.
high-altitude
pulmonary e. (HAPE)
idiopathic cyclic e.
interstitial e.
interstitial pulmonary e.
myocardial e.
neurogenic pulmonary e.
periorbital e.
peripheral e.
postanesthesia
pulmonary e.

postcardioversion
pulmonary e.
pulmonary e.
**edge**
e. detection
leading e.
trailing e.
**edrophonium chloride**
**EDV**
end-diastolic volume
**Edwards catheter**
**EEG**
electroencephalogram
**EF**
ejection fraction
**effect**
Anrep e.
Bainbridge e.
band saw e.
Compton e.
Doppler e.
erectile e.
inotropic e.
jet e.
neurotoxic e.
Rivero-Carvallo e.
snowplow e.
training e.
Venturi e.
Wedensky e.
Windkessel e.
**effective**
e. arterial elastance (Ea)
e. balloon dilating area
(EBDA)
**efficiency**
detective quantum e.
**effort**
e. angina
e. syndrome
e. thrombosis
**effusion**
pericardial e.
pleural e.

**effusive-constrictive pericarditis**
**E to F slope**
**Eggleston method**
**Ehlers-Danlos syndrome**
**Ehret's phenomenon**
**eicosapentaenoic acid**
*Eikenella corrodens*
**Einthoven's**
    E. equation
    E. law
    E. triangle
**Eisenmenger reaction**
**Eisenmenger's**
    E. complex
    E. disease
    E. physiology
    E. syndrome
    E. tetralogy
**ejection**
    e. click
    e. fraction (EF)
    e. fraction systolic
    e. murmur
    e. period
    e. phase
    e. phase index
    e. rate
    e. shell image
    e. sound
    e. time
    e. velocity
**ejection-fraction image**
**Ejrup maneuver**
**EKG**
    electrocardiogram
**EKY**
    electrokymogram
**Elantan**
**elastance**
    effective arterial e. (Ea)
    end-systolic e.
**elastic**
    e. component
    e. lamina

    e. stiffness
    e. tissue hyperplasia
**elasticity**
**elasticum**
    pseudoxanthoma e.
**Elastorc catheter guide wire**
**Elavil**
**elbow flexion**
**ELCA**
    excimer laser coronary
    angioplasty
**Elecath**
    E. circulatory support
    device
    E. switch box
**elective cardioversion**
**electrical**
    e. ablation
    e. activation abnormality
    e. alternans
    e. alternation of heart
    e. axis
    e. cardioversion
    e. countershock
    e. disease
    e. failure
    e. fulguration
    e. hazard
    e. heart position
    e. injury
**electric cardiac pacemaker**
**electrocardiogram (ECG, EKG)**
    unipolar e.
**electrocardiographic**
    e. complex
    e. wave
    e. wave complex (QRS
    complex)
**electrocardiography**
    ambulatory e.
    esophageal e.
    exercise e.
    fetal e.

**electrocardiography** *(continued)*
    intracardiac e.
    12-lead e.
**electrocardiophonogram**
**electrocardiophonography**
**electrochemical polarization**
**electroconvulsive therapy**
**electrode**
    AE-60-I-2 implantable
     pronged unipolar e.
    AE-85-I-2 implantable
     pronged unipolar e.
    AE-60-KB implantable
     unipolar endocardial e.
    AE-85-KB implantable
     unipolar endocardial e.
    AE-60-K-10 implantable
     unipolar endocardial e.
    AE-85-K-10 implantable
     unipolar endocardial e.
    AE-60-KS-10 implantable
     unipolar endocardial e.
    AE-85-KS-10 implantable
     unipolar endocardial e.
    bipolar myocardial e.
    e. catheter
    central terminal e.
    dispersing e.
    epicardial e.
    exploring e.
    hydrogen e.'s
    implantable
     cardioverter e.'s
    indifferent e.
    e. jelly
    Lifeline e.
    monopolar temporary e.
    MVE-50 implantable
     myocardial e.
    Myowire cardiac e.
    Myowire II cardiac e.
    Nyboer esophageal e.
    pacemaker e.'s
    e. paddle

    PE-60-I-2 implantable
     pronged unipolar e.
    PE-85-I-2 implantable
     pronged unipolar e.
    PE-60-KB implantable
     unipolar endocardial e.
    PE-85-KB implantable
     unipolar endocardial e.
    PE-60-K-10 implantable
     unipolar endocardial e.
    PE-85-K-10 implantable
     unipolar endocardial e.
    PE-85-KS-10 implantable
     unipolar endocardial e.
    reference e.
    silent e.
    Skylark surface e.
    Stockert cardiac
     pacing e.
    Surgicraft pacemaker e.
    e. system
    transvenous e.
**electrode-skin interface**
**electroencephalogram (EEG)**
**electroencephalography**
**electrogram**
    coronary sinus e.
    His bundle e.
**electrokymogram (EKY)**
**electrokymograph**
**electrokymography**
**electrolyte**
    e. imbalance
**electromanometer**
**electromechanical**
    e. coupling
    e. dissociation
    e. interval
    e. systole
**electronic**
    e. distance compensation
    e. fetal monitor
    e. pacemaker load
    e. scanning

electron volt
electrophoresis
electrophysiologic
    e. mapping
    e. study (EPS)
    e. test
electrophysiology
    intracardiac e.
electrostethograph
electrosurgery
Elema leads
element
    contractile e.
    series elastic e.
elevation
    ST segment e.
elfin facies
El Gamal coronary bypass
  catheter
elimination half-life
Elite pacemaker
ellipse
    prolate e.
elliptical loop
Ellis-van Creveld syndrome
embolectomy
    catheter e.
    e. catheter
    femoral e.
    pulmonary e.
emboli
embolic
    e. abscess
    e. aneurysm
    e. pneumonia
    e. stroke
embolism
    air e.
    amniotic fluid e.
    aortic e.
    atheroma e.
    atheromatous e.
    bland e.
    cellular e.

cholesterol e.
coronary e.
crossed e.
direct e.
fat e.
gas e.
hematogenous e.
infective e.
miliary e.
multiple e.
obturating e.
oil e.
pantaloon e.
paradoxical e.
plasmodium e.
pulmonary e.
pyemic e.
retrograde e.
riding e.
saddle e.
straddling e.
submassive pulmonary e.
tumor e.
venous e.
embolization
    air e.
    cholesterol e.
    coil e.
    paradoxical e.
    septic e.
    e. therapy
    transcatheter e.
embolized foreign material
embolomycotic aneurysm
embolotherapy
embolus, pl. emboli
    air e.
    catheter e.
    cerebral e.
    femoral e.
    paradoxical e.
    saddle e.
embryocardia
    jugular e.

**embryologic**
**embryology**
**emergency**
    e. care
    hypertensive e.
    e. reperfusion
**Emery-Dreifuss**
    E.-D. disease
    E.-D. muscular
      dystrophy
**emesis**
**emetine toxicity**
**Eminase**
**emission**
    single-photon e.
**emotional stress**
**emphysema**
**empiric constant**
**empyema**
    e. of pericardium
    pulsating e.
**emulsion**
    intravascular
      perfluorochemical e.
**enalapril**
    e. maleate
**enalaprilat**
**encainide**
    e. hydrochloride
**Encapsulon**
    E. epidural catheter
    E. sheath introducer
    E. vessel dilator
**encarditis**
**encephalomyocarditis**
**encephalopathy**
    hypertensive e.
    metabolic e.
**encircling endocardial
ventriculotomy**
**Encor pacemaker**
**encrustation theory of
atherosclerosis**

**end**
    distal e.
    proximal e.
**endarterectomy**
    blunt eversion carotid e.
    carotid e.
    coronary e.
    femoral e.
**endarteritis**
**end-diastolic**
    e.-d. count
    e.-d. dimension
    e.-d. left ventricular
      pressure
    e.-d. pressure
    e.-d. volume (EDV)
**end-hole #7 French catheter**
**endoauscultation**
**endocardiac, endocardial**
**endocardiography**
**endocarditic**
**endocarditis**
    abacterial thrombotic e.
    acute bacterial e.
    atypical verrucous e.
    bacteria-free stage of
     bacterial e.
    bacterial e.
    cachectic e.
    e. chordalis
    constrictive e.
    culture-negative e.
    fungal e.
    gram-negative e.
    *Haemophilus* e.
    infectious e., infective e.
    isolated parietal e.
    Libman-Sacks e.
    Löffler's e., Löffler's
     fibroplastic e.
    malignant e.
    marantic e.
    mitral valve e.
    mural e.

nonbacterial
thrombotic e.
nonbacterial verrucous e.
e. parietalis fibroplastica
polypous e.
prosthetic valve e.
rheumatic e.
septic e.
subacute bacterial e.
(SBE)
terminal e.
ulcerative e.
valvular e.
vegetative e.,
verrucous e.
**endocardium**
**endocrine**
e. disorder
e. system
**endocytosis**
**endogenous lipid**
**endomyocardial**
e. biopsy
e. disease
e. fibroelastosis
e. fibrosis
**endomyocarditis**
**endonuclease**
restriction e.
**endopericarditis**
**endoperimyocarditis**
**endoperoxide steal**
**endophthalmitis**
**endorphin**
**endothelial-derived relaxant factor**
**endothelium**
**endotracheal intubation**
**endpoint**
therapeutic e.
**end-pressure artifact**
**endralazine**
**end-stage renal disease**

**end-systolic**
e.-s. count
e.-s. dimension
e.-s. elastance
e.-s. left ventricular
pressure
e.-s. pressure
e.-s. pressure-volume
relation
e.-s. stress-dimension
relation
e.-s. volume (ESV)
**Enduron**
**enema**
barium e.
Kayexalate e.
sodium polystyrene
sulfonate e.
**energy**
e. production
e. resolution
e. supply
**enhancement**
leading edge e.
**Enkaid**
**enlargement**
cardiac e.
left atrial e.
right atrial e. (RAE)
**enoximone**
**entangling technique**
**enteric**
e. cytopathogenic human
orphan virus (ECHO
virus)
e. fistula
**enteric-coated aspirin**
**enterovirus**
**entoptic pulse**
**entrainment of tachycardia**
**entrance**
e. block
e. wound
**entry site**

*ERBE cryotherapy* (handwritten)

**enzyme**
  allosteric modification of e.
  angiotensin-converting e. (ACE inhibitor, ACE)
  cardiac e.
  lysosomal e.
  proteolytic e.
**eosinophil**
**eosinophilia**
**eosinophilic pneumonia**
**Epanutin**
**ephedrine**
**epicardial**
  e. electrode
  e. fat
  e. lead
**epicardium**
**epidermal growth factor**
**epidural anesthesia**
**epilepsy**
**epinephrine**
**epistaxis**
**e point**
**E point-septal separation (EPSS)**
**epoprostenol sodium**
**Eppendorf catheter**
**EPS**
  electrophysiologic study
**EPSS**
  E point-septal separation
**Epstein-Barr virus**
**equation**
  continuity e.
  Doppler e.
  Doppler continuity e.
  Einthoven's e.
  Ford e.
  Gorlin e.
  Holen-Hatle e.
  Nernst e.
  regression e.
  Rodrigo e.

  Starling e.
  Torricelli's orifice e.
**equilibrium**
  voltage e.
**equiphasic complex**
**equivalency**
  left main e.
**equivalent**
  anginal e.
  metabolic e. (MET)
  right anterior oblique e.
**erbium:YAG laser**
**Erb's atrophy**
**Erdheim disease**
**erectile effect**
**ergometry**
  bicycle e.
**ergonovine**
  e. maleate
  e. provocation test
  e. test
**ergot alkaloid**
**ergotamine**
**erosion**
  spark e.
**eruptive xanthoma**
*Erysipelothrix*
**erythema**
  e. marginatum
  e. multiforme
**erythematosus**
  lupus e.
  pericarditis of systemic lupus e.
  systemic lupus e. (SLE)
**erythrityl tetranitrate**
**erythrocyte sedimentation rate (ESR)**
**erythrocytosis**
**erythroderma**
**erythrogenin**
**erythromycin**
**erythropheresis**

**escape**
    e. beat
    e. impulse
    e. interval
    junctional e. beat
    nodal e.
    e. rhythm
    ventricular e.
**escape-capture bigeminy**
**escaped**
    e. beat
    e. contraction
    e. ventricular
    contraction
*Escherichia coli*
**Esidrix**
**E sign**
**Esimil**
**Esmarch tourniquet**
**esmolol hydrochloride**
**esophageal**
    e. cardiogram
    e. echocardiography
    e. electrocardiography
    e. lead
    e. reflux
    e. rupture
    e. spasm
**esophagitis**
    peptic e.
    reflux e.
**esophagus**
    Barrett's e.
**ESR**
    erythrocyte sedimentation
    rate
**essential**
    e. bradycardia
    e. hypertension
    e. tachycardia
**EST**
    exercise stress test
**ester**
    cholesterol e.

**Estes point system**
**estrogen**
**ESV**
    end-systolic volume
**ESWL**
    extracorporeal shock wave
    lithotripsy
**ETCO2 multigas analyzer**
**ethacrynic acid**
**ethambutol**
    e. hydrochloride
**ethanol**
**ether test**
**Ethibond suture**
**Ethmozine**
**ethyl alcohol**
**ethylenediaminetetraacetic acid**
  **disodium salt**
**etiologic diagnosis**
**etiology**
**etomidate**
**etoposide**
**European Coronary Surgery**
  **Study**
**eustachian valve**
**eusystole**
**eusystolic**
**euthyroid sick syndrome**
**evaluation**
    laboratory e.
    noninvasive e.
**event**
    cerebral e.
    cerebrovascular e.
    intracardiac e.
    e. recorder
**eversion**
    blunt e.
    cusp e.
**evolving myocardial infarction**
**Ewart's sign**
**Ewing's sign**
**examination**
    apical e.

**examination** *(continued)*
    cardiac e.
    funduscopic e.
    neurologic e.
    parasternal e.
    physical e.
    supraclavicular e.
    suprasternal e.
**excavatum**
    pectus e.
**exchange**
    gas e.
    e. guide wire
    pulmonary gas e.
    sodium-potassium e.
**excimer**
    e. laser
    e. laser coronary
      angioplasty (ECLA,
      ELCA)
**excisional cardiac surgery**
**excitability**
    supranormal e.
**excitable gap**
**excitation**
    premature e.
    supernormal e.
**excitation-contraction coupling**
**exclusion criteria**
**excretion**
**excursion**
    dome e.
**exercise**
    ankle e.
    e. capacity
    dynamic e.
    e. echocardiography
    e. electrocardiography
    e. factor
    e. index
    e. intolerance
    isometric e.
    isotonic e.
    e. regimen

    e. scintigraphy
    strenuous e.
    e. stress test (EST)
    e. study
    supine e.
    e. test
    e. tolerance test
    e. treadmill
    upright e.
**exercise-induced silent myocardial ischemia**
**exertion**
    perceived e.
**exertional**
    e. angina
    e. dyspnea
**exfoliative dermatitis**
**exit**
    e. block
    e. wound
**Exna**
**exocardia**
**exocardial murmur**
**exogenous lipid**
**exon**
**exophthalmos**
**expansion**
    infarct e.
**expectancy**
    life e.
**expectoration**
**experiment**
    Müller's e.
    Weber's e.
**expert**
    e. system
    e. testimony
**expired air collection**
**exploring electrode**
**exposure**
    chemical e.
    cold e.
    toxin e.

**extension**
 infarct e.
 knee e.
 Linx guide wire e.
**external**
 e. cardiac massage
 e. carotid artery
 e. defibrillator
 e. grid
 e. jugular vein
 e. mammary artery
 e. pacemaker
**extracardiac**
 e. murmur
 e. shunt
**extracorporeal**
 e. circulation
 e. membrane oxygenator
 e. pump oxygenator
 e. shock wave
  lithotripsy (ESWL)
**extraction**
 lactate e.
 e. reserve

**extrarenal azotemia**
**extrasystole**
 atrial e.
 atrioventricular e., A-
  V e.
 atrioventricular nodal e.,
  A-V nodal e.
 auricular e.
 AV junctional e.
 infranodal e.
 interpolated e.
 junctional e.
 lower nodal e.
 midnodal e.
 nodal e.
 return e.
 supraventricular e.
 upper nodal e.
 ventricular e.
**extremity ischemia**
**eyeless needle**

**Fab** fragments
**Fabry's** disease
**facial** vein
**facies**, pl. **facies**
    aortic f.
    Corvisart's f.
    elfin f.
    mitral f.
**facioscapulohumeral**
    f. dystrophy
    f. dystrophy of
      Landouzy-Déjérine
**factor**
    atrial natriuretic f.
     (ANF)
    basic fibroblastic
     growth f. (BFGF)
    behavioral f.
    coagulation f.
    duty f.
    endothelial-derived
     relaxant f.
    epidermal growth f.
    exercise f.
    fibroblast growth f.
    gravitation f.
    growth f.
    Hageman f.
    insulin-like growth f.
     (IGF)
    f. IX
    myocardial depressant f.
     (MDF)
    necrosis f.
    f. P
    platelet-derived growth f.
    psychological f.
    psychosocial f.
    rheumatoid f.
    risk f.
    tissue f.

    transforming growth f.
     (TGF)
    tumor necrosis f. (TNF)
    f. VIII
    von Willebrand f.
    f. X
**failure**
    acute renal f.
    acute respiratory f.
     (ARF)
    backward heart f.
    cardiac f.
    chronic renal f.
    circulatory f.
    congestive heart f.
     (CHF)
    coronary f.
    electrical f.
    forward heart f.
    heart f.
    hepatic f.
    high-output heart f.
    left ventricular f.
    low-output heart f.
    myocardial f.
    pacemaker f.
    power f.
    pulmonary f.
    pump f.
    renal f.
    right heart f.
    right-sided heart f.
    right ventricular f.
**fainting**
    hysterical f.
    f. lark
**faintness**
**Fallot**
    tetralogy of F.
**Fallot's**
    F. pentalogy
    F. tetrad

**Fallot's** *(continued)*
   F. tetralogy
   F. triad
**false**
   f. aneurysm
   f. angina
   f. aortic aneurysm
   f. dextrocardia
   f. tendon
**familial**
   f. abetalipoproteinemia
   f. amyloidosis
   f. dysautonomia
   f. hypercholesterolemia
   f. hypertrophic
    obstructive
    cardiomyopathy
   f. nephritis
**far field**
**FAS**
   fetal alcohol syndrome
**fascial layer**
**fascicular**
   f. beat
   f. block
   f. heart block
**fast channel**
**FAST right heart**
  **cardiovascular catheter**
**fat**
   body f.
   dietary f.
   f. embolism
   epicardial f.
   f. pulmonary embolism
**fatty**
   f. acid
   f. heart
   f. streak
**F-18 2-deoxyglucose (FDG)**
**FDG**
   F-18 2-deoxyglucose
   2-fluoro-2-deoxyglucose
**felodipine**

**female hormone**
**femoral**
   f. approach
   f. arteriography
   f. artery
   f. artery occlusion
   f. artery thrombosis
   f. embolectomy
   f. embolus
   f. endarterectomy
   f. perfusion cannula
   f. vascular injury
   f. vein
   f. vein occlusion
   f. venous thrombosis
   f. vessel
**femoropopliteal, femoral-**
  **popliteal**
   f. bypass
   f. bypass graft
   f. graft
**femorotibial**
   f. bypass
   f. bypass graft
   f. graft
**fenestration**
   aortopulmonary f.
**fenofibrate**
**fenoldopam**
**fenoldopam mesylate**
**fentanyl**
**Fergie needle**
**Ferguson needle**
**ferritin**
**fetal**
   f. alcohol syndrome
    (FAS)
   f. bradycardia
   f. circulation
   f. electrocardiography
   f. heart rate
   f. tachycardia
**fetus**

**fever**
    acute rheumatic f.
     (ARF)
    hemorrhagic f.
    Q f.
    relapsing f.
    rheumatic f.
    Rocky Mountain
     spotted f.
    scarlet f.
    typhoid f.
    yellow f.
**FFP**
    fresh frozen plasma
**F gate**
**fiber**
    atriohisian f.'s
    His-Purkinje f.'s
    James f.'s
    Kent f.'s
    Mahaim f.'s
    f. optic catheter delivery
     system
    Purkinje f.'s
    f. shortening
    terminal Purkinje f.'s
**fiberoptic**
    f. catheter
    f. oximeter catheter
**fibric acid**
**fibrillary waves**
**fibrillation**
    atrial f., auricular f.
    paroxysmal atrial f.
    f. threshold
    ventricular f.
**fibrin**
    f. split product
    f. thrombus
**fibrinogen degradation product**
**fibrinogen-fibrin degradation**
  **product**
**fibrinoid degeneration**
**fibrinolysis**

**fibrinolytic**
    f. reaction
    f. system
    f. therapy
**fibrinopeptide A**
**fibrinous pericarditis**
**fibrin-specific antibody**
**Fibriscint**
**fibroblast growth factor**
**fibroelastoma**
    papillary f.
**fibroelastosis**
    endocardial f.,
     endomyocardial f.
**fibroma**
**fibromuscular dysplasia**
**fibromusculoelastic lesion**
**fibronectin**
**fibroplastic**
    f. cardiomyopathy
    f. disease
**fibroplastica**
    endocarditis parietalis f.
**fibrosarcoma**
**fibrosis**
    annulus f.
    biventricular
     endomyocardial f.
    cystic f.
    endocardial f.
    endomyocardial f.
    progressive interstitial
     pulmonary f.
    pulmonary f.
    tropical
     endomyocardial f.
**fibrosum**
    pericardium f.
**fibrotic**
**fibrous**
    f. body
    f. dysplasia
    f. dysplasia of bone
    f. plaque

**fibrous** *(continued)*
    f. skeleton
    f. subaortic stenosis
**Fick**
    F. cardiac output
    F. method
    F. oxygen method
    F. principle
    F. technique
**Fiedler's myocarditis**
**field**
    far f.
    near f.
    f. of view
**fight-or-flight**
    f.-o.-f. reaction
    f.-o.-f. response
**figure-of-eight abnormality**
**figure-of-eight suture**
**filariasis**
**filiform pulse**
**filling**
    diastolic f.
    ventricular f.
**film**
    density-exposure
      relationship of f.
    f. density-exposure
      relationship
    f. developer
    drying f.
    f. drying
    f. fixer bath
    f. processing
    serial cut f.'s
    f. viewer
    f. wash bath
**filming**
    serialographic f.
**filter**
    arterial f.
    Bird's Nest vena
      caval f.
    BTF-37 arterial blood f.

    Gianturco-Roehm Bird's
      Nest vena cava f.
    Greenfield f.
    Interface arterial
      blood f.
    Jostra arterial blood f.
    Kimray-Greenfield f.
    K-37 pediatric arterial
      blood f.
    Mobin-Uddin f.
    Mobin-Uddin vena
      cava f.
    Simon Nitinol inferior
      vena cava f.
    Swank high-flow arterial
      blood f.
    William Harvey arterial
      blood f.
**filtration**
    x-ray beam f.
**final rapid repolarization**
**finger dilation**
**Finochietto retractor**
**first**
    f. degree A-V block
    f. degree heart block
    f. heart sound ($S_1$)
    f. obtuse marginal
      artery (OM-1)
    f. shock count
    f. third filling fraction
**first-order kinetics**
**first-pass radionuclide**
  **angiocardiography**
**Fischer's symptom**
**fish-mouth**
    f.-m. incision
    f.-m. mitral stenosis
**fish oil**
**fistula**, pl. **fistulae, fistulas**
    aortocaval f.
    arteriovenous f.
    carotid-cavernous f.
    coronary artery f.

coronary artery-right
  ventricular f.
enteric f.
pulmonary
  arteriovenous f.
renal f.
subclavian
  arteriovenous f.
traumatic f.

**Fitch obturator**
**fitness**
biological f.
cardiovascular f.

**five-chamber view**
**fixed**
f. coupling
f. rate mode
f. rate pulse generator

**fixed-rate pacemaker**
**fixer bath**
**FK-506**
**flail mitral valve**
**flap**
intimal f.

**flash-lamp excited pulsed dye**
**Flaxedil**
**flea-bitten kidney**
**flecainide**
**flexibility**
**flexion**
elbow f.
hip f.
shoulder f.
shoulder horizontal f.
trunk forward f.

**Flint's murmur**
**Flolan**
**floppy**
f. guide wire
f. mitral valve
f. tip guide wire
f. valve syndrome

**Florex medical compression**
  **stockings**

**flosequinan**   TIMI II

**flow**
f. across orifice
arterial blood f.
f. artifact
blood f.
blood f. measurement
cerebral blood f. (CBF)
coronary blood f. (CBF)
f. injector
laminar f.
laminar blood f.
f. mapping
pulmonary blood f.
pulsatile f.
f. rate
f. ratio (Qp/Qs)
systemic blood f. (SBF)
transvalvular f.
tricuspid valve f.
f. velocity

**flow-directed**
f.-d. balloon
  cardiovascular catheter
f.-d. catheter

**flucytosine**
**fluid**
f. aspiration
crystalloid f.
f. dynamics
f. mechanics
pericardial f.
pleural f.

**fluid-filled catheter**
**Fluitran**
**flumazenil**
**flunarizine**
**fluorescein angiography**
**fluorescence-guided "smart"**
  **laser**
**fluorescence spectroscopy**
**fluoride toxicity**
**fluorine-18**
**fluorocarbon poisoning**

5-fluorocytosin
2-fluoro-2-deoxyglucose (FDG)
**fluorography**
  spot-film f.
**fluoroscopic**
  f. calcium
  f. guidance
  f. visualization
**fluoroscopy**
  biplane f.
**Fluosol**
**fluoxetine**
**flurazepam**
**flushed**
  aspirated and f.
**flush technique**
**flutter**
  atrial f., auricular f.
  atrial fibrillation f.
  diaphragmatic f.
  impure f.
  ventricular f.
**flutter-fibrillation**
  f.-f. waves
**fluvastatin**
**fluxionary hyperemia**
**foam**
  f. cell
  gel f.
  polyurethane f.
**focal block**
**Fogarty**
  F. calibrator
  F. catheter
  F. embolectomy catheter
**fold**
  bulboventricular f.
**folic acid**
**Fontan's procedure**
**foot ulcer**
**foramen, pl. foramina**
  bulboventricular f.
  interventricular f.
  f. ovale, oval f.

**force**
  left ventricular f.'s
  peak twitch f.
  Starling f.'s
**forced**
  f. beat
  f. cycle
**force-frequency relation**
**force-length relation**
**forceps**
  Adson f.
  biopsy f.
  coagulation f.
  Cook flexible biopsy f.
  DeBakey tissue f.
  Rumel thoracic f.
**force-velocity-length relation**
**force-velocity relation**
**force-velocity-volume relation**
**Ford equation**
**foreign body**
**form**
  wave f.
**format**
  quad screen f.
  scanning f.
**formation**
  impulse f.
**formula, pl. formulas, formulae**
  Bazett's f.
  biplane f.
  Cannon's f.
  Gorlin f.
  Hakki f.
  Poiseuille's resistance f.
**Forney's syndrome**
***fortuitum***
  *Mycobacterium f.*
**forward**
  f. conduction
  f. heart failure
  f. triangle technique
**fosinopril sodium**
**fossa, pl. fossae**

antecubital f.
f. ovalis
supraclavicular f.
**four-chamber view**
**Fourier**
F. analysis
F. series analysis
F. transform
F. transform analysis
**fourth heart sound ($S_4$)**
**foveated chest**
**fraction**
ejection f., ejection f.
  systolic (EF)
first third filling f.
global left ventricular
  ejection f.
left ventricular
  ejection f. (LVEF)
MB f.
regurgitant f.
right ventricular
  ejection f. (RVEF)
shortening f.
**fractional**
f. myocardial shortening
f. shortening
**fragment**
catheter f.
Fab f.'s
**fragmentation**
f. myocarditis
f. of myocardium
**Framingham Heart Study**
**Frank lead system**
**Frank-Starling**
F.-S. curve
F.-S. mechanism
**Frank-Straub-Wiggers-Starling**
  **principle**
**Fräntzel's murmur**
**Franzen needle guide**
**Fraunhofer zone**

**fremitus**
friction f.
pericardial f.
**French**
F. double lumen
  catheter
F. JR4 Schneider
  catheter
F. SAL catheter
F. shaft catheter
F. sheath
F. size
F. sizing of catheter
**frequency**
dynamic f. response
fundamental f.
natural f.
resonant f.
f. response
**fresh frozen plasma (FFP)**
**Fresnel zone**
**friction**
f. fremitus
f. murmur
f. rub
f. sound
**friction rub**
pericardial f. r.
**Friedreich's**
F. ataxia
F. disease
F. sign
**front wall needle**
**frosted heart**
**Frumil**
**fucosidosis**
**fugax**
amaurosis f.
**fulguration**
electrical f.
**fully automatic pacemaker**
**fulminans**
purpura f.

**function**
>atrial transport f.
>cardiac f.
>cardiovascular f.
>contractile f.
>f. curve
>diastolic f.
>hepatic f.
>left ventricular f.
>lung f.
>mitochondrial f.
>myocardial f.
>parasympathetic f.
>pulmonary f.
>pump f.
>renal f.
>respiratory f.
>right ventricular f.
>sinus node f.
>systolic f.
>ventricular f.

**functional**
>f. assessment
>f. classification

>f. congestion
>f. dyspnea
>f. image
>f. imaging
>f. murmur
>f. pain
>f. subtraction

**fundamental frequency**
**fundus,** pl. **fundi**
**funduscopic examination**
**fungal**
>f. endocarditis
>f. infection

**fungus,** pl. **fungi**
**funnel dynamics**
**furosemide**
**fusiform**
>f. aneurysm
>f. aortic aneurysm

**fusion**
>f. beat
>commissural f.

**F wave**
**f wave**

**Ga**
    gallium
**$^{68}$Ga**
    gallium-68
**gain**
    g. control
    time compensation g. (TCG)
    time-varied g. (TVG)
**Gairdner's disease**
**Gaisböck's syndrome**
**galactosidase deficiency**
**Galaxy pacemaker**
**Gallagher bipolar mapping probe**
**gallamine triethiodide**
**Gallavardin's phenomenon**
**gallbladder disease**
**gallium (Ga)**
**gallium-68 ($^{68}$Ga)**
**gallop**
    atrial g.
    presystolic g.
    protodiastolic g.
    g. rhythm
    $S_4$ g.
    $S_3$ g.
    g. sound
    summation g.
    systolic g.
**gallopamil**
*gambiense*
    *Trypanosoma g.*
**gamma**
    g. camera
    g. globulin
    g. ray
**ganglion**
    stellate g.
**ganglionic blocker**
**gangliosidosis**

**gangrene**
    gas g.
**gap**
    auscultatory g.
    excitable g.
    g. junction
    g. phenomenon
    silent g.
**gargoylism**
**garment**
    antishock g.
    pneumatic antishock g.
**Garrett dilator**
**Gärtner's**
    G. method
    G. tonometer
    G. vein phenomenon
**gas**
    g. clearance
    g. clearance measurement
    g. clearance method
    g. constant (R)
    g. embolism
    g. exchange
    g. gangrene
**gaseous pulse**
**gases**
    arterial blood g.
    blood g.
**gastrocardiac syndrome**
**gastroepiploic artery**
**gastroesophageal reflux**
**gastrointestinal**
    g. symptom
    g. tract
**gate**
    d g.
    F g.
    h g.
    m g.

**gated**
>g. blood pool scanning
>g. computed tomography
>g. list mode
>g. system

**gating**
>in-memory g.
>g. mechanism

**Gaucher's disease**

**gauge**
>strain g.

**Gc protein**

**GDP**
>guanosine 5'-diphosphate

**gel**
>aluminum hydroxide g.
>g. foam

**gemfibrozil**

**Gen2 pacemaker**

**general anesthesia**

**generator**
>asynchronous pulse g.
>atrial synchronous pulse g.
>atrial triggered pulse g.
>Coratomic implantable pulse g.
>demand pulse g.
>fixed rate pulse g.
>Maxilith pacemaker pulse g.
>Medtronic pulse g.
>Microlith pacemaker pulse g.
>Minilith pacemaker pulse g.
>pulse g.
>standby pulse g.
>Stilith implantable cardiac pulse g.
>ventricular inhibited pulse g.
>ventricular synchronous pulse g.
>ventricular triggered pulse g.
>Vivalith II pulse g.
>x-ray g.

**gene secretor**

**genetic**
>g. counseling
>g. disorder
>g. heterogeneity
>g. hypertrophic cardiomyopathy
>g. locus
>g. transmission

**genetics**

**genin**

**Gensini**
>G. catheter
>G. coronary arteriography catheter

**gentamicin**

**geometry of stenosis**

**gerontology**

**gestational hypertension**

**ghost vessel**

**giant**
>g. cell aortitis
>g. cell arteritis
>g. cell myocarditis

**Gianturco coil**

**Gianturco-Roehm Bird's Nest vena cava filter**

**Gianturco-Roubin stent**

**Gibson murmur**

**GISSI**
>Gruppo Italiano Per lo Studio Della Streptokinase Nell'Infarto Miocardio

**gitalin**

**giving-up-given-up response**

*glabrata*
>*Torulopsis g.*

**gland**
>adrenal g.
>parathyroid g.

pituitary g.
prostate g.
thyroid g.

**glare**
veiling g.
**Glasgow's sign**
**Glattelast compression pantyhose**
**Glenn shunt**
**Glenn's operation**
**global left ventricular ejection fraction**
**Global Utilization of Streptokinase and TPA for Occluded Coronary Arteries protocol (GUSTO protocol)**
**globular thrombus**
**globulin**
antilymphocyte g.
antithymocyte g.
gamma g.
**glomerulonephritis**
acute g. (AGN)
**glossopharyngeal neuralgia**
**glucagon**
**glucocorticoid**
**glucocorticosteroid**
**gluconate**
calcium g.
potassium g.
quinidine g.
**glucose**
g. intolerance
g. metabolism
g. uptake
**glucose-6-phosphate dehydrogenase**
**glucose-insulin-potassium**
**glucose-6-phosphatase**
**glucosidase deficiency**
**glutamate**
**glutamic-oxaloacetic transaminase (GOT)**
**glutethimide**

**glyceraldehyde 3-phosphate**
**glycerol**
**glyceryl trinitrate**
**glycogen**
g. cardiomegaly
g. phosphorylase
g. storage disease
g. storage disease of heart
g. synthase
**glycogenosis**
cardiac g.
**glycolysis**
**glycopyrrolate**
**glycoside**
cardiac g.
digitalis g.
**glycosis**
**glycosphingolipid disorder**
**glycyrrhizinic acid**
**Glyrol**
**GMP**
guanosine monophosphate
**goiter**
**Golaski-UMI vascular prosthesis**
**gold (Au)**
**Goldblatt's**
G. hypertension
G. phenomenon
**gold-195m**
**Goldman risk-factor index**
**gonadal**
g. disease
g. dysgenesis
g. hormone
**Goodale-Lubin catheter**
**gooseneck deformity**
*gordonae*
*Mycobacterium* g.
**Gore-Tex**
G.-T. cardiovascular patch
G.-T. surgical membrane

**Gore-Tex** *(continued)*
    G.-T. tube
    G.-T. vascular graft
**Gorlin**
    G. catheter
    G. constant
    G. equation
    G. formula
**Gorlin's syndrome**
**GOT**
   glutamic-oxaloacetic
   transaminase
**Gott shunt**
**gout**
**Gowers'**
    G. contraction
    G. sign
    G. syndrome
**grabbing technique**
**gracile habitus**
**gradient**
    aortic pressure g.
    aortic valve g.
    atrioventricular g.
    Doppler pressure g.
    intracavitary pressure g.
    mitral g.
    mitral valve g. (MVG)
    peak systolic g. (PSG)
    peak transaortic valve g.
    (AVG)
    pressure g.
    pulmonary valve g.
    g. reduction
    residual g.
    systolic g.
    transaortic valve g.
    ventricular g.
**grading**
**graft**
    aortofemoral bypass g.
    aortoiliac bypass g.
    bypass g.

    coronary artery
     bypass g. (CABG)
    Dacron g.
    femoropopliteal g.
    femorotibial g.
    Gore-Tex vascular g.
    Impra-Graft microporous
     PTFE vascular g.
    lower extremity
     bypass g.
    mammary artery g.
    mesenteric bypass g.
    Microknit patch g.
    Poly-Plus Dacron
     vascular g.
    renal artery bypass g.
    saphenous vein g.
    Shiley Tetraflex
     vascular g.
    skip g.
    subclavian artery
     bypass g.
    Varivas R denatured
     homologous vein g.
    vein g.
    Velex woven Dacron
     vascular g.
    vertebral artery
     bypass g.
    Vitagraft vascular g.
**Graham**
    G. Steell's murmur
**gram-negative**
    g.-n. endocarditis
    g.-n. pericarditis
**granular cell tumor**
**granulocytopenia**
**granuloma**
    sarcoid g.
**granulomatosis**
    allergic g.
    lymphomatoid g.
    Wegener's g.
**granulomatous arteritis**

graphic record
Gräupner's method
Graves disease
gravidarum
    chorea g.
    hyperemesis g.
gravis
    myasthenia g.
gravitation factor
gray scale
great
    g. artery
    g. vessel
Greenfield filter
grid
    external g.
grievance protocol
griseofulvin
Grocco's sign
Grollman
    G. catheter
    G. pulmonary artery
    seeking catheter
Grönblad-Strandberg syndrome
groove
    bulboventricular g.
    conoventricular fold
    and g.
    terminal g.
growth
    g. factor
    g. hormone
    g. retardation
Grüntzig
    G. catheter
    G. femoral stiffening
    cannula
    G. technique
Gruppo Italiano Per lo Studio
Della Streptokinase
Nell'Infarto Miocardio
(GISSI)

GTP
    guanosine 5'-triphosphate
guanabenz
guanadrel
guanethidine monosulfate
guanethidine sulfate
guanfacine
guanosine 5'-diphosphate
    (GDP)
guanosine monophosphate
    (GMP)
guanosine 5'-triphosphate
    (GTP)
guidance
    echo g.
    fluoroscopic g.
guide
    ACS LIMA g.
    Franzen needle g.
    movable core straight
    safety wire g.
    Slidewire extension g.
    tapered movable core
    curved wire g.
    Tefcor movable core
    straight wire g.
    wire g.
    g. wire
guider
    NL3 g.
guiding catheter
Guillain-Barré syndrome
gunshot wound
GUSTO protocol
    Global Utilization of
    Streptokinase and TPA for
    Occluded Coronary
    Arteries protocol
guttural pulse
gynecomastia

habitus
  gracile h.
**hadow balloon**
*Haemophilus*
  *H. haemolyticus*
  *H. influenzae*
*Haemophilus* **endocarditis**
**Hageman factor**
**hairy heart**
**Hakki formula**
**Hakko Dwelicath catheter**
**half amplitude pulse duration**
**half-life**
  biological h.-l.
  elimination h.-l.
**half-power distance**
**Halfprin**
**half-time**
  pressure h.-t.
**half-value layer**
**Hall-Kaster**
  H.-K. prosthetic valve
  H.-K. valve
**halogenated**
  h. hydrocarbon
  h. hydrocarbon
  propellant
**haloperidol**
**halo sheathing**
**halothane**
**Halsted clamp**
**hamartoma**
**Hamman-Rich syndrome**
**Hamman's**
  H. disease
  H. sign
**Hampton's hump**
**Hancock**
  H. bipolar balloon
  pacemaker
  H. embolectomy catheter
  H. fiberoptic catheter

  H. hydrogen detection
  catheter
  H. luminal
  electrophysiologic
  recording catheter
  H. temporary cardiac
  pacing wire
  H. wedge-pressure
  catheter
**handgrip**
  isometric h.
**Hand-Schüller-Christian**
  **disease**
**hanging heart**
**hangout interval**
**HAPE**
  high-altitude pulmonary
  edema
**hard pulse**
**harmonic content**
**Harris adapter**
**Hartmann clamp**
**Hartzler**
  H. balloon catheter
  H. dilatation catheter
**hazard**
  electrical h.
**HCl**
  hydrochloride
**HDFP**
  Hypertension Detection and
  Follow-Up Program
**HDL**
  high-density lipoprotein
**headache**
  migraine h.
  syncopal migraine h.
**head-hunter catheter**
**heart**
  air-driven artificial h.
  armored h.
  artificial h.

**heart** *(continued)*
  athlete's h.
  athletic h.
  h. attack
  h. beat
  beer h.
  h. block
  bony h.
  boot-shaped h.
  contour of h.
  crisscross h.
  dilatation of h.
  h. disease
  disordered action of h.
   (DAH)
  drop h.
  h. failure
  fatty h.
  frosted h.
  glycogen storage disease
   of h.
  hairy h.
  hanging h.
  Holmes h.
  horizontal h.
  hypoplastic h.
  hypoplastic left h.
  icing h.
  intermediate h.
  irritable h.
  Jarvik-7 artificial h.
  left h.
  h. loop
  luxus h.
  movable h.
  h. murmur
  parchment h.
  pendulous h.
  Penn State h.
  h. position
  pulmonary h.
  h. rate (HR)
  h. rate reserve
  h. reflex

  right h.
  sabot h.
  semihorizontal h.
  semivertical h.
  septation of h.
  skin h.
  soldier's h.
  h. sound
  Starling's law of the h.
  stone h.
  h. stroke
  superoinferior h.
  suspended h.
  swinging h.
  systemic h.
  Taussig-Bing h.
  teardrop h.
  tiger h.
  tobacco h.
  total artificial h.
  h. transplant
  transverse section of h.
  h. tube
  univentricular h.
  upstairs-downstairs h.
  Utah artificial h.
  h. valve
  venous h.
  vertical h.
  wandering h.
  water-bottle h.
  wooden-shoe h.
**heartbeat**
**heart failure**
  congestive h. f. (CHF)
  diastolic h. f.
  forward h. f.
  systolic h. f.
**heart-forming region (HFR)**
**heart-lung**
  h.-l. bypass
  h.-l. machine
  h.-l. transplant

**heat**
    h. load
    h. stroke
**Heath-Edwards criteria**
**heatstroke**
**heave**
**heavy metal**
**Heberden's angina**
**Hegglin's syndrome**
**Heim-Kreysig sign**
**Heimlich maneuver**
**helices**
**helicopter**
    Life Flight h.
**helium-cadmium diagnostic laser**
**helix, pl. helices**
    amphipathic h.
**Helix PTCA dilatation catheter**
**helminthic myocarditis**
**hemadostenosis**
**hemangioendothelioma**
**hemangioma**
**hemangiomatosis**
**hemangiosarcoma**
**Hemaquet sheath**
**Hemashield**
**hematocrit**
**hematogenous embolism**
**hematologic disease**
**hematoma**
    aneurysmal h.
    dissecting h.
**hematoporphyrin derivative (HPD)**
**hematuria**
**hemautogram**
**hemiazygos vein**
**hemiblock**
    left anterior h. (LAH)
    left middle h.
    left posterior h.
    left septal h.

**hemicardia**
**hemic murmur**
**hemisystole**
**hemitruncus**
**hemochromatosis**
**hemoclip**
**hemodialysis**
**hemodilution**
**hemodynamic**
    h. abnormality
    h. assessment
    h. collapse
    h. maneuver
    h. principle
    h. tolerance
    h. vise
**hemodynamic-angiographic study**
**hemodynamics**
    intraoperative h.
    systemic h.
**hemofiltration**
**hemoglobin**
**hemoglobin-oxygen dissociation curve**
**hemolytic anemia**
**hemoperfusion**
**hemopericardium**
***Hemophilus***
**hemopneumopericardium**
**hemoptysis**
    cardiac h.
**hemopump**
**hemorheology**
**hemorrhage**
    reperfusion-induced h.
    splinter h.
**hemorrhagic**
    h. fever
    h. telangiectasia
**hemosiderosis**
    pulmonary h.
    transfusional h.
**hemostasis valve**

hemostat
    Kelly h.
    Mayo h.
    mosquito h.
    straight h.
hemothorax
Henle's
    H. elastic membrane
    H. loop
    H. tenestrated
      membrane
Henoch-Schönlein
    H.-S. purpura
    H.-S. syndrome
Henry-Gauer response
heparin
heparin-coated guide wire
heparin-dihydroergotamine
heparinization
heparinized saline
hepatic
    h. disease
    h. failure
    h. function
    h. lipase
    h. vein
    h. vein catheterization
hepatitis
    h. B
    h. C
    viral h.
hepatojugular
    h. reflux
    h. reflux test
hepatomegaly
hepatosplenomegaly
hereditary
    h. ataxia
    h. hemorrhagic
      telangiectasia
heredity
heredopathia atactica
    polyneuritiformis

hernia
    hiatal h.
    inguinal h.
    umbilical h.
heroin
herpes zoster
herzstoss
Hespan
heterogeneity
    genetic h.
heterograft
    porcine h.
heterologous cardiac
    transplantation
heterometric autoregulation
*Heterophyes*
heterophyiasis
heterotaxia
    cardiac h.
heterotopic cardiac
    transplantation
heterozygosity
heterozygote
Hexabrix
hexaxial reference system
hexosaminidase deficiency
HFR
    heart-forming region
Hg
    mercury
$^{195m}$Hg
    mercury-195m
h gate
hiatal hernia
hibernating myocardium
hibernation
    myocardial h.
high
    h. altitude
    h. blood pressure
    h. fiber diet
high-altitude pulmonary edema
    (HAPE)
high-density lipoprotein (HDL)

high-flow catheter
high-molecular-weight dextran
high-output heart failure
high-risk
    h.-r. angioplasty
    h.-r. patient
high-torque wire
hilar dance
Hill's
    H. phenomenon
    H. sign
Hi-Per
    H.-P. Flex exchange
    wire
    H.-P. Flex wire
hip flexion
His
    H. bundle
    bundle of H.
    H. bundle electrogram
    H. spindle
His-Purkinje
    H.-P. fibers
    H.-P. system
    H.-P. tissue
histamine
histiocytoma
histocompatibility agent B27
histogram mode
*Histoplasma*
histoplasmic pericarditis
histoplasmosis
His-ventricular (H-V)
Hi-Torque
    H.-T. floppy exchange
    guide wire
    H.-T. floppy with
    Propel
    H.-T. intermediate guide
    wire
HIV
    human immunodeficiency
    virus
    HIV cardiomyopathy

HLA
    human lymphocyte antigen
HLHS
    hypoplastic left heart
    syndrome
hoarseness
Hodgkin's disease
Hodgkin-Huxley
    H.-H. constant
    H.-H. model
Hodgkin-Key murmur
Hodgson's disease
holder
    Björk-Shiley heart
    valve h.
    blade control wire h.
    Castroviejo needle h.
    catheter h.
    catheter guide h.
    needle h.
    Watson heart value h.
    wire h.
Holen-Hatle equation
holiday heart syndrome
holism
Hollenhorst plaque
Holmes heart
holmium laser
holodiastolic
holosystolic murmur
Holter monitor
Holt-Oram syndrome
Homans' sign
homeometric autoregulation
*hominis*
    *Cardiobacterium h.*
homocystinuria syndrome
homogentisic acid oxidase
   deficiency
homograft
    aortic h.
homologous cardiac
   transplantation
homozygosity

**homozygote**
**honk**
    precordial h.
    systolic h.
**hook**
    barbed h.
    Bryant mitral h.
**Hopkins aortic clamp**
**Horizon surgical ligating and marking clip**
**horizontal heart**
**hormone**
    adrenocorticotropic h. (ACTH)
    antidiuretic h. (ADH)
    female h.
    gonadal h.
    growth h.
    natriuretic h.
    parathyroid h.
    thyroid h.
    thyroid-stimulating h.
**Horton's arteritis**
**hose**
    Juzo h.
**hospital-acquired infection**
**hospital information system**
**hot spot**
**hot-tip laser probe**
**hourglass**
    h. murmur
    h. pattern
**HPD**
    hematoporphyrin derivative
**H-Q interval**
**HR**
    heart rate
**H-R conduction time**
**5HT**
    5-hydroxytryptamine
**hub**
    catheter h.
**Hufnagel**
    H. aortic clamp

    H. ascending aortic clamp
**Hughes-Stovin syndrome**
**Hull's triad**
**hum**
    cervical venous h.
    venous h.
**human**
    h. catheterization technique
    h. coronary angiography technique
    h. immunodeficiency virus (HIV)
    h. lymphocyte antigen (HLA)
    h. lymphocyte antigen typing
    h. menopausal gonadotropin coenzyme A reductase inhibitor
**humeroperoneal neuromuscular disease**
**humidity**
**hump**
    Hampton's h.
**Humulin insulin**
**Hunter detachable balloon occluder**
**Hunter's**
    H. operation
    H. syndrome
**Hunter-Satinsky clamp**
**Huntington's chorea**
**Hurler-Scheie compound**
**Hurler's syndrome**
**Hürthle manometer**
**H-V**
    His-ventricular
    H-V conduction time
    H-V interval
**h wave**
**hyaline thrombus**
**hybrid unit**

hydatid cyst
hydralazine
hydraulic resistance
hydrazine
    dimethyl h.
Hydrenox
hydrobromide
    hydroxyamphetamine h.
hydrocarbon
    halogenated h.
    h. toxicity
hydrochloride (HCl)
    clonidine h.
    desipramine h.
    diltiazem h.
    doxepin h.
    encainide h.
    esmolol h.
    ethambutol h.
    meperidine h.
    mepivacaine h.
    methoxamine h.
    metoclopramide h.
    mexiletine h.
    mitoxantrone h.
    naloxone h.
    nortriptyline h.
    phenoxybenzamine h.
    phentolamine h.
    phenylephrine h.
    prazosin h.
    prenalterol h.
    procainamide h.
    procaine h.
    propranolol h.
    protriptyline h.
    sotalol h.
    terazosin h.
    tetracaine h.
    thioridazine h.
    tolazoline h.
    trazodone h.
hydrochlorothiazide

hydrocortisone
    h. sodium succinate
hydrocyanic acid
HydroDIURIL
hydroflumethiazide
hydrogen
    h. density
    h. electrodes
    h. peroxide
Hydromox
hydronephrosis
hydropericarditis
hydropericardium
hydrophilic coated guide wire
hydropneumopericardium
hydrops pericardii
hydrosphygmograph
Hydro-T
hydrothorax
hydroxyamphetamine
    hydrobromide
hydroxychloroquine sulfate
18-hydroxycorticosterone
hydroxyethyl starch
17-hydroxylase deficiency
hydroxyl radical
3-hydroxy-3-methylglutaryl
    coenzyme A reductase
3-hydroxy-3-methylglutaryl
    coenzyme A reductase
    inhibitor
5-hydroxytryptamine (5HT)
hydroxyurea
hydroxyzine
Hygroton
Hylorel
Hypaque
Hypaque-76
hyperabduction syndrome
hyperaldosteronism
hyperalimentation
hyperalphalipoproteinemia
hyperbaric pressure
hypercalcemia

hypercalciuria
hypercapnia
hypercardia
hyperchloremic acidosis
hypercholesterolemia
    familial h.
hyperchylomicronemia
hypercontractility
hypercyanotic
    h. angina
    h. spell
hyperdiastole
hyperdicrotic
hyperdicrotism
hyperdynamic
    h. apex cardiogram
    h. state
hyperemesis gravidarum
hyperemia
    active h.
    arterial h.
    collateral h.
    fluxionary h.
    passive h.
    peristatic h.
    reactive h.
    venous h.
hyperemic
hypereosinophilia
hypereosinophilic syndrome
hyperestrogenemia
hypergammaglobulinemia
hyperglycemia
hyperkalemia
hyperkinemia
hyperkinesis
hyperkinetic
    h. heart syndrome
    h. pulse
    h. state
hyperlipidemia
    multiple lipoprotein-
        type h.
hyperlipoproteinemia

hypermagnesemia
hypernatremia
hypernephroma
hyperoxaluria
hyperparathyroidism
hyperphosphatemia
hyperpiesis, hyperpiesia
hyperpietic
hyperplasia
    adrenal h.
    bilateral adrenal h.
    congenital adrenal h.
    elastic tissue h.
    intimal h.
hypersensitive carotid sinus
    syndrome
hypersensitivity
    aminosalicylic acid h.
    carotid sinus h.
    h. myocarditis
    h. pneumonitis
    h. vasculitis
hypersphyxia
Hyperstat
hypersystole
hypersystolic
hypertension
    accelerated-malignant h.
    adrenal h.
    benign h.
    borderline h.
    diastolic h.
    essential h.
    gestational h.
    Goldblatt's h.
    idiopathic h.
    labile h.
    left atrial h.
    malignant h.
    orthostatic h.
    pale h.
    pediatric h.
    portal h.
    postpartum h.

pregnancy-induced h.
primary h.
primary pulmonary h.
pulmonary h.
renal h.
renoprival h.
renovascular h.
salt-and-water
  dependent h.
systemic h.
systolic h.
venous h.
**Hypertension Detection and
  Follow-Up Program (HDFP)**
**hypertensive**
  h. arteriopathy
  h. arteriosclerosis
  h. crisis
  h. emergency
  h. encephalopathy
  h. hypertrophic
    cardiomyopathy
  h. pulmonary vascular
    disease
  h. retinopathy
  h. urgency
**hyperthermia**
**hyperthyroidism**
  amiodarone-induced h.
  apathetic h.
**hypertriglyceridemia**
**hypertrophic**
  h. cardiomyopathy
  h. obstructive
    cardiomyopathy
  h. pulmonary
    osteoarthropathy
**hypertrophy**
  asymmetric h.
  asymmetric septal h.
  cardiac h.
  compensatory h. of
    heart

concentric left
  ventricular h.
left ventricular h.
  (LVH)
lipomatous h.
myocardial h.
right ventricular h.
  (RVH)
septal h.
ventricular h.
volume load h.
**hyperuricemia**
**hyperuricemic nephropathy**
**hyperventilation maneuver**
**hyperviscosity syndrome**
**hypervitaminosis**
**hypervitaminosis D**
**hypervolemia**
**hypervolemic**
**hyphemia**
**hypnosis**
**hypnotic**
**hypoalbuminemia**
**hypoaldosteronism**
  hyporeninemic h.
**hypoalphalipoproteinemia**
**hypocalcemia**
**hypocholesterolemia**
**hypochondriasis**
**hypodynamia**
  h. cordis
**hypofunction**
**hypoglossal nerve**
**hypoglycemia**
**hypoglycemic**
  h. agent
  h. syncope
**hypokalemia**
**hypokinemia**
**hypokinesis, hypokinesia**
**hypokinetic pulse**
**hypomagnesemia**
**hyponatremia**
**hypoparathyroidism**

**hypophosphatemia**
**hypopiesis**
    orthostatic h.
**hypoplasia**
    mitral valve h.
    right ventricular h.
**hypoplastic**
    h. heart
    h. left heart
    h. left heart syndrome
    (HLHS)
**hyporeninemia**
**hyporeninemic**
  hypoaldosteronism
**hyposphyxia**
**hypostasis**
**hypostatic congestion**
**hyposystole**
**hypotension**
    arterial h.
    orthostatic h.
    postural h.
    vasovagal h.
**hypotensive**
**hypothermia**
    moderate h.
**hypothesis**
    leading circle h.
    lipid h.
    Lyon h.
    monoclonal h.
    response-to-injury h.

**hypothyroidism**
**hypotonia**
**hypotonicity**
**hypotonus, hypotony**
**Hypovase**
**hypoventilation**
    alveolar h.
**hypovolemia**
**hypovolemic shock**
**hypoxanthine**
**hypoxemia**
    arterial h.
    h. test
**hypoxia**
    altitude h.
    alveolar h.
    hypoxic h.
    ischemic h.
    stagnant h.
**hypoxic**
    h. hypoxia
    h. spell
    h. syncope
**hysteresis**
    pacing h.
**hysterical**
    h. fainting
    h. syncope
**hysterosystole**
**H zone**

**IABP**
    intra-aortic balloon pump
**iatrogenic**
    i. atrial septal defect
    i. disorder
**ibopamine**
**ibuprofen**
**ice-pick view**
**icing heart**
**ictometer**
**ictus cordis**
**idiojunctional rhythm**
**idionodal rhythm**
**idiopathic**
    i. bradycardia
    i. cardiomegaly
    i. cardiomyopathy
    i. cyclic edema
    i. dilated
      cardiomyopathy
    i. dilation
    i. hypertension
    i. hypertrophic subaortic
      stenosis (IHSS)
    i. restrictive
      cardiomyopathy
    i. thrombocytopenic
      purpura
**idioventricular**
    i. kick
    i. rhythm
**IGF**
    insulin-like growth factor
**IHSS**
    idiopathic hypertrophic
      subaortic stenosis
**iliac**
    i. artery
    i. artery occlusion
    i. steal
    i. vein
    i. vein thrombosis

**image**
    amplitude i.
    ejection-fraction i.
    ejection shell i.
    functional i.
    i. intensifier
    paradox i.
    parametric i.
    phase i.
    T1 weighted i.
    T2 weighted i.
**imaging**
    acoustic i.
    i. biplane
    blood pool i.
    i. chain
    dipyridamole-thallium i.
    functional i.
    krypton-81m
      ventilation i.
    magnetic resonance i.
      (MRI)
    mask-mode cardiac i.
    myocardial i.
    myocardial perfusion i.
    nuclear magnetic
      resonance i.
    platelet i.
    pyrophosphate i.
    radionuclide i.
    spin echo i.
    stress thallium-201
      myocardial perfusion i.
    i. study
    $^{99m}$Tc i.
    technetium-99m i.
    thallium i.
    thallium perfusion i.
    video i.
    xenon lung ventilation i.

**imbalance**
    acid-base i.
    electrolyte i.
**IMED infusion pump**
**imipenem**
**imipramine**
**immunoassay**
    nifedipine enzyme i.
**immunoglobulin**
**immunological theory**
**immunosuppressive therapy**
**immunotherapy**
**impedance**
    acoustic i.
    aortic i.
    arterial i.
    atrial lead i.
    i. catheter
    i. modulus
    pacemaker i.
    i. plethysmography
    vascular i.
**imperfecta**
    osteogenesis i.
**implantable**
    i. cardioverter-
        defibrillator
    i. cardioverter electrodes
**implantation**
**Impra-Graft microporous
    PTFE vascular graft**
**impulse**
    afferent i.
    apex i.
    cardiac i.
    i. conduction
    ectopic i.
    escape i.
    i. formation
    point of maximum i.
        (PMI)
    i. propagation
    i. summation
    systolic apical i.

**impure flutter**
$^{111}$**In**
    indium-111
**inactivity**
    physical i.
**incessant tachycardia**
**incidence**
    peak i.
**incident**
    vascular i.
**incision**
    fish-mouth i.
    median sternotomy i.
    stab i.
    thoracotomy i.
    transverse i.
**incisura apicis cordis**
**incisura pulse**
**incompetence, incompetency**
    aortic i.
    cardiac i.
    mitral i.
    muscular i.
    pulmonary i.,
        pulmonic i.
    pyloric i.
    relative i.
    tricuspid i.
    valvular i.
**incomplete**
    i. atrioventricular
        dissociation
    i. A-V dissociation
**incontinentia pigmenti
    syndrome**
**incremental atrial pacing**
**Indacrinone**
**indapamide**
**indecainide**
**Inderal**
**Inderal-LA**
**index**, gen. **indicis**, pl. **indices**,
    **indexes**
    ankle/brachial i.

atherectomy i.
body mass i. (BMI)
brachial/ankle i.
cardiac i. (CI)
cardiac output i.
cardiac risk i.
diastolic pressure-time i.
  (DPTI)
eccentricity i.
ejection phase i.
exercise i.
Goldman risk-factor i.
isovolumetric phase i.
isovolumic i.
left atrial emptying i.
left ventricular diastolic
  phase i.
mitral valve closure i.
oxygen consumption i.
ponderal i.
pulmonary vascular
  resistance i.
Quetelet i.
relaxation time i.
risk i.
Robinson i.
segmental pressure i.
shock i.
stroke i.
stroke work i.
systemic vascular
  resistance i.
systolic pressure-time i.
tension-time i.
i. value
vascular resistance i.
**indicator dilution technique**
**indifferent electrode**
**indirect**
  i. diuretic
  i. lead
**indium-111 ($^{111}$In)**
**indocyanine**
  i. green

i. green dye
i. green indicator
  dilution technique
i. green method
**indomethacin**
**indoramin**
**induration**
  brown i. of lung
**indurative myocarditis**
**indwelling line**
**infantile beriberi**
**infarct**
  i. avid myocardial
    scintigraphy
  brain i.
  i. expansion
  i. extension
  lacunar i.
**infarction**
  acute myocardial i.
    (AMI)
  anterior myocardial i.
  anteroinferior
    myocardial i.
  anterolateral
    myocardial i.
  anteroseptal
    myocardial i.
  atrial i.
  cardiac i.
  cerebral i.
  completed myocardial i.
  diaphragmatic
    myocardial i.
  evolving myocardial i.
  inferior myocardial i.
  inferior wall
    myocardial i. (IWMI)
  inferolateral
    myocardial i.
  intestinal i.
  lateral myocardial i.
  myocardial i. (MI)
  myocardial i. in H-form

**infarction** *(continued)*
    non-Q-wave
      myocardial i.
    nontransmural
      myocardial i. (NTMI)
    posterior myocardial i.
    postmyocardial i.
    pulmonary i.
    recurrent myocardial i.
    right ventricular i.
    silent myocardial i.
    subacute myocardial i.
    subendocardial
      myocardial i.
    thrombolysis and
      angioplasty in
      myocardial i. (TAMI)
    through-and-through
      myocardial i.
    transmural myocardial i.
    watershed i.
**infected**
    i. aneurysm
    i. myxoma
**infection**
    bacterial i.
    community-acquired i.
    fungal i.
    hospital-acquired i.
    respiratory i.
    spirochetal i.
    staphylococcal i.
    streptococcal i.
    systemic i.
**infectious**
    i. endocarditis
    i. mononucleosis
**infective**
    i. embolism
    i. endocarditis
    i. pericarditis
**inferior**
    i. mesenteric vascular
    occlusion

    i. myocardial infarction
    i. vena cava (IVC)
    i. vena cava occlusion
    i. wall myocardial
      infarction (IWMI)
**inferolateral myocardial**
  **infarction**
**infiltrative cardiomyopathy**
**inflammatory reaction**
**inflation**
    balloon i.
**inflow tract**
**influenza**
*influenzae*
    Haemophilus i.
**informed consent**
**infracristal**
**infradiaphragmatic portion**
**infranodal extrasystole**
**infrared-pulsed laser**
**infrarenal abdominal aortic**
  **aneurysm**
**Infrasonics ventilator**
**infundibular**
    i. obstruction
    i. stenosis
**infundibular stenosis**
**infundibulectomy**
**infundibulum**
**infusion**
    nitroprusside i.
**inguinal hernia**
**inhalation**
    i. agent
    oxygen i.
**Inhibace**
**inhibited pacing**
**inhibition**
    potassium i.
**inhibitor**
    ACE i.
    angiotensin-converting
    enzyme

acyl cholesterol
  acyltransferase i.
carbonic anhydrase i.
converting enzyme i.
cyclooxygenase i.
human menopausal
  gonadotropin coenzyme
  A reductase i.
3-hydroxy-3-
  methylglutaryl
  coenzyme A
  reductase i.
MAO i.
    monoamine oxidase
      inhibitor
  monoamine oxidase i.
    (MAO inhibitor)
  oxysterol i.
  phosphodiesterase i.
  $\alpha_2$-plasmin i.
  plasminogen activator i.
  renin i.
  thromboxane
    synthetase i.
**in-hospital cardiac arrest**
**injection**
  bolus i.
**injector**
  flow i.
  power i.
  pressure i.
**injury**
  blunt i.
  diastolic current of i.
  electrical i.
  femoral vascular i.
  median nerve i.
  myocardial i.
  penetrating i.
  reperfusion i.
  systolic current of i.
  vascular i.
**in-memory gating**

**innocent**
  i. murmur
  i. murmur of elderly
**innominate artery**
**Innovace**
**Innovar**
**Inocor**
**inorganic murmur**
**inosine**
**inotropic**
  i. agent
  i. effect
**inotropy**
**Inoue**
  I. balloon
  I. balloon catheter
  I. self-guiding balloon
**insect sting**
**insertion**
  percutaneous catheter i.
  retrograde catheter i.
  route of i.
  wire i.
**inspiratory dyspnea**
**instability**
  catheter i.
**instantaneous**
  i. electrical axis
  i. vector
**instrument**
  arterial oscillator
    endarterectomy i.
  Matsuda titanium
    surgical i.'s
  Wolvek sternal
    approximation
    fixation i.
**instrumentation**
  angiographic i.
**insudate**
**insufficiency**
  aortic i.
  aortic valvular i.
  arterial i.

**insufficiency** *(continued)*
    atrioventricular valve i.
    cardiac i.
    cerebrovascular i.
    coronary i.
    mitral i.
    myocardial i.
    pulmonary i.
    pulmonic i.
    renal i.
    rheumatic mitral i.
    tricuspid i.
    valvular i.
    venous i.
**insulin**
    beef i.
    Humulin i.
    Lente i.
    NPH i.
    pork i.
**insulin-like growth factor (IGF)**
**intellectual dysfunction**
**intensifier**
    image i.
**intensity**
    spatial i.
**intensive care**
**interatrial**
    i. baffle
    i. conduction
    i. septum
**intercadence**
**intercadent**
**intercalary**
**intercept angle**
**interdependence**
    ventricular i.
**interectopic interval**
**interface**
    electrode-skin i.
**Interface arterial blood filter**

**interference**
    i. beat
    i. dissociation
**interlaced scanning**
**intermediary vesicle**
**intermediate**
    i. heart
    i. syndrome
**intermediate-density lipoprotein**
**Intermedics RES Q implantable cardioverter-defibrillator**
**intermittence, intermittency**
**intermittent**
    i. claudication
    i. coronary sinus occlusion
    i. pneumatic compression
    i. positive pressure breathing (IPPB)
    i. pulse
**internal**
    i. adhesive pericarditis
    i. carotid artery
    i. diameter
    i. jugular vein
    i. mammary artery
    i. mammary artery graft angiography
**internodal**
    i. conduction
    i. pathways
**interpolated extrasystole**
**interrupted aortic arch**
**interruption**
    aortic arch i.
**intersegmental arteries**
**Intersept cardiotomy reservoir**
**interstitial**
    i. edema
    i. pulmonary edema
    i. space
**intersystole**

**intersystolic period**
**interval**
> A-H i.
> A-N i.
> atriocarotid i., a-c i.
> atrio-Hisian i.
> A-V i.
> B-H i.
> cardioarterial i., c-a i.
> coupling i.
> electromechanical i.
> escape i.
> hangout i.
> H-Q i.
> H-V i.
> interectopic i.
> isometric i.
> magnet pacing i.
> P-A i.
> passive i.
> P-J i.
> postsphygmic i.
> P-P i.
> P-Q i.
> P-R i.
> presphygmic i.
> Q-R i.
> Q-RB i.
> QRS i.
> Q-S$_2$ i.
> Q-T i.
> R-R i.
> sphygmic i.
> systolic time i.'s (STI)
> V-A i.

**interval-strength relation**
**intervention**
**interventional**
> i. cardiac catheterization
> i. catheterization
> i. echocardiography
> i. study

**interventricular**
> i. foramen

**i. septal motion**
> i. septal motion
> i. septal rupture
> i. septum
> i. septum aneurysm
> i. sulcus
> i. veins

**intervertebral disk**
**intestinal**
> i. infarction
> i. ischemia
> i. lipodystrophy

**intestine**
**intima**
**intimal**
> i. flap
> i. hyperplasia
> i. tear

**Intimax vascular catheter**
**intolerance**
> carbohydrate i.
> exercise i.
> glucose i.

**intoxication**
> alcohol i.
> digitalis i.

**intra-aortic**
> i.-a. balloon
> i.-a. balloon catheter
> i.-a. balloon device
> i.-a. balloon pump
> (IABP)

**intra-arterial**
> i.-a. counterpulsation

**intra-atrial**
> i.-a. baffle
> i.-a. block
> i.-a. conduction
> i.-a. conduction time

**intracardiac**
> i. catheter
> i. electrocardiography
> i. electrophysiologic
> study
> i. electrophysiology

**intracardiac** *(continued)*
    i. event
    i. lead
    i. mass
    i. pacing
    i. pressure
    i. pressure curve
    i. shunt
    i. sucker
    i. thrombus
**intracaval device**
**intracavitary pressure gradient**
*intracellulare*
    Mycobacterium i.
**intracoronary thrombolysis balloon valvuloplasty**
**intraluminal**
**intramural coronary arteries**
**intramyocardial pressure**
**intraoperative**
    i. hemodynamics
    i. mapping
**intrapericardial pressure**
**intrathoracic pressure**
**intrauterine echocardiography**
**intravascular**
    i. foreign body retrieval
    i. perfluorochemical emulsion
    i. pressure
    i. stent
    i. ultrasound (IVUS)
    i. volume
**intravenous**
**intraventricular**
    i. aberration
    i. block
    i. conduction
    i. conduction delay
    i. conduction pattern
    i. septum
**Intrepid balloon catheter**
**intrinsic**
    i. deflection

    i. sympathomimetic activity (ISA)
**intrinsicoid deflection**
**introducer**
    Angestat hemostasis i.
    Angetear tearaway i.
    Cardak percutaneous catheter i.
    Encapsulon sheath i.
    Razi cannula i.
    i. sheath
    Tuohy-Bost i.
    UMI transseptal Cath-Seal catheter i.
    USCI i.
**Intropin**
**intubation**
    endotracheal i.
    tracheal i.
**invalidism**
**invasive**
    i. assessment
    i. pressure measurement
**inversion**
    population i.
    ventricular i.
**inversus**
    situs i.
**inverted T-waves**
**inward-going rectification**
**iodide**
    metocurine i.
**iodine**
**iohexol**
**ion**
    calcium i.
    chloride i.
    potassium i.
    sodium i.
**Ionescu-Shiley pericardial patch**
**iopamidol**
**ioversol**

**ioxaglate**
    i. meglumine
    i. sodium
    sodium meglumine i.
**IPPB**
    intermittent positive
    pressure breathing
**iron storage disease**
**irregularly irregular pulse**
**irreversible shock**
**irritable heart**
**ISA**
    intrinsic sympathomimetic
    activity
**ischemia**
    brachiocephalic i.
    cardiac i.
    cerebral i.
    colonic i.
    exercise-induced silent
      myocardial i.
    extremity i.
    intestinal i.
    limb i.
    mesenteric i.
    myocardial i.
    silent i.
    silent myocardial i.
    subendocardial i.
    transient i.
**ischemic**
    i. cardiomyopathy
    i. contracture of left
      ventricle
    i. heart disease
    i. hypoxia
    i. myocardium
    i. paralysis
**ISIS-2**
    Second International Study
    of Infarct Survival
**Ismelin**
**ISMO, Ismo**
**isocenter system**

**isochoric**
**isodiphasic complex**
**isoelectric**
    i. line
    i. period
    i. point
**isoenzyme**
**isoetharine**
**isoflurane**
**isoform**
**isolated**
    i. dextrocardia
    i. parietal endocarditis
**isometric**
    i. contraction
    i. exercise
    i. handgrip
    i. interval
    i. period
    i. period of cardiac
      cycle
**isoniazid**
**isonitrile**
    carbomethoxyisopropyl i.
    methoxyisobutyl i.
**Isopaque**
**isoproterenol stress test**
**Isoptin**
**isorhythmic dissociation**
**isosorbide**
    i. dinitrate
    i. mononitrate
**isotonic**
    i. contraction
    i. exercise
**isotope**
**isovolume**
**isovolumetric**
    i. phase index
    i. relaxation
**isovolumic**
    i. index
    i. relaxation
    i. relaxation period

**Isovue**
**isozyme**
> myocardial muscle creatine kinase i. (CK-MB)

**isradipine**
*israelii*
> *Actinomyces i.*
> *Nocardia i.*

**Isuprel**
**IVAC infusion pump**

**Ivalon plug**
**I-V block**
**IVC**, pl. **venae cavae**
> inferior vena cava

**IVT percutaneous catheter introducer sheath**
**IVUS**
> intravascular ultrasound

**IWMI**
> inferior wall myocardial infarction

**J**
> joule

**Jacobson**
> J. microbulldog clamp
> J. modified vessel
> clamp

**Jacobson-Potts clamp**

**James**
> J. fibers
> J. tracts

**Janeway lesion**

**Jarvik-7 artificial heart**

**Jatene's procedure**

**Javid**
> J. bypass clamp
> J. carotid artery bypass
> clamp
> J. carotid artery clamp

**j curve**

**jejunal artery**

**jelly**
> electrode j.

**Jenkins Activity Survey**

**jeopardy score**

**Jervell and Lange-Nielsen
syndrome**

**jet**
> j. effect
> residual j.

**J-exchange wire**

**J-guide wire**

**joint deformity**

**Jones criteria**

**Josephson**
> J. catheter
> J. quadpolar catheter

**Jostra**
> J. arterial blood filter
> J. cardiotomy reservoir
> J. catheter

**joule (J)**

**J point**

**JR4 catheter**

**JR5 catheter**

**J Rosen guide wire**

**J-tip**
> J.-t. guide wire

**Judkins**
> J. catheter
> J. coronary catheter
> J. guiding catheter
> J. technique
> J. torque control
> catheter

**Judkins-Sones technique of
cardiac catheterization**

**jugular**
> j. embryocardia
> j. pulse
> j. vein
> j. venous distention
> (JVD)
> j. venous pressure
> j. venous pulse
> j. venous pulse tracing

**jumping thrombosis**

**junction**
> atrioventricular j.
> gap j.
> loose j.
> QRS-ST j.
> ST j.
> tight j.
> triadic j.

**junctional**
> atrioventricular j.
> tachycardia
> j. beat
> j. complex
> j. escape beat
> j. escape rhythm
> j. extrasystole
> j. rhythm

**juvenile**
- j. arrhythmia
- j. pattern
- j. rheumatoid arthritis

**juxtaductal coarctation**

**Juzo hose**

**JVD**
- jugular venous distention

**j wire**

**K-37 pediatric arterial blood filter**
**kallikrein**
**kallikrein-bradykinin system**
**Kallmann's syndrome**
**Kantrowitz thoracic clamp**
**Kaon**
**Kaopectate**
**Kaplan Meier survival curve**
**Kaposi's sarcoma**
**Kartagener's**
 K. syndrome
 K. triad
**Katz-Wachtel phenomenon**
**Kawai bioptome**
**Kawasaki's disease**
**Kay balloon**
**Kayexalate enema**
**Kay-Shiley caged-disc valve**
**K current**
**Kearns-Sayre syndrome**
**Kearns' syndrome**
**Keith's bundle**
**Kelly**
 K. clamp
 K. hemostat
**Kelly-Wick vascular tunneler**
**Kensey catheter**
**Kent fibers**
**Kent's bundle**
**Kerley**
 K. A line
 K. B line
**Keshan disease**
**ketamine**
**keV**
 kiloelectron volt
**kick**
 atrial k.
 idioventricular k.
**kidney**
 Ask-Upmark k.

 flea-bitten k.
 polycystic k.
**Kifa catheter material**
**Killip classification**
**kiloelectron volt (keV)**
**kilovolt (kV)**
**Kimray-Greenfield filter**
**kinase**
 creatine k. (CK)
 phosphorylase k.
 protein k.
**kinetics**
 first-order k.
 zero-order k.
**kinetocardiogram**
**kinetocardiograph**
**King**
 K. ASD umbrella closure
 K. bioptome
 K. double umbrella closure system
***kingae***
 *Kingella k.*
***Kingella kingae***
**King's biopsy method**
**kinin**
**kininogen**
**kinked aorta**
**Kisch's reflex**
**kissing balloon technique**
**kit**
 neonatal internal jugular puncture k.
 percutaneous catheter introducer k.
 thermodilution k.
 thermodilution catheter introducer k.
***Klebsiella pneumoniae***
**Klinefelter's syndrome**
**Klippel-Feil syndrome**

**Klippel-Trenaunay-Weber
syndrome**
**knee extension**
**knife**, pl. **knives**
    Lebsche sternal k.
    valvotomy k.
    k. wound
**knob**
    aortic k.
**knock**
    pericardial k.
**knuckle**
    b k.
    cervical aortic k.
    k. sign
**Koch's triangle**
**Konno**
    K. biopsy method
    K. bioptome
    K. operation
**Kontron**
    K. balloon
    K. intra-aortic balloon
    pump

**Korotkoff's sound**
**$^{81m}$Kr**
    krypton-81m
**Kreysig's sign**
**Krönig's steps**
**krypton-8lm ventilation
imaging**
**krypton-81m ($^{81m}$Kr)**
**Kugelberg-Welander**
    K.-W. disease
    K.-W. syndrome
**Kugel's artery**
**Kussmaul's**
    K. paradoxical pulse
    K. sign
    K. symptom
**kV**
    kilovolt
**kwashiorkor**
**kymogram**
**kymography**
**kymoscope**
**kyphoscoliosis**

labetalol
labile hypertension
Laboratories
    Venereal Disease
    Research L. (VDRL)
laboratory
    l. evaluation
    l. testing
lactate
    amrinone l.
    l. dehydrogenase
    l. extraction
    Ringer's l.
    l. threshold
lactic
    l. acid
    l. acid dehydrogenase
*Lactobacillus*
lacunar infarct
LAD, pl. arteries
  left axis deviation
  left anterior descending
  artery
ladder diagram
LAH
  left anterior hemiblock
laid-back view
LAMB
  lentigines, atrial myxoma,
    mucocutaneous myxomas,
    and blue nevi
  LAMB syndrome
Lambert-Kay clamp
lamina
    elastic l.
laminar
    l. blood flow
    l. flow
laminated
    l. clot
    l. thrombus
lanatoside C

Lancisi's sign
Landolfi's sign
Landouzy-Déjérine
    L.-D. dystrophy
    facioscapulohumeral
     dystrophy of L.-D.
    L.-D. syndrome
Lanoxicaps
Lanoxin
LAO
  left anterior oblique
  LAO position
Laplace relationship
Laplace's law of heart
large-vessel disease
lark
    fainting l.
larva migrans
    ocular l. m.
    visceral l. m.
laryngeal
    l. nerve
    l. vertigo
laser
    l. ablation
    l. angioplasty
    argon l.
    atheroblation l.
    balloon-centered argon l.
    erbium:YAG l.
    excimer l.
    fluorescence-guided
     "smart" l.
    helium-cadmium
     diagnostic l.
    holmium l.
    infrared-pulsed l.
    l. light
    microsecond pulsed
     flashlamp pumped
     dye l.
    Nd:YAG l.

**laser** *(continued)*
    neodymium:yttrium-
      aluminum-garnet laser
    neodymium:yttrium-
      aluminum-garnet l.
      (Nd:YAG laser,
      Nd:YAG laser)
    rotational ablation l.
    spectroscopy-directed l.
    Surgilase 150 l.
    XeCl l.
    XeCl excimer l.
    xenon chloride l. (XeCl
    laser)
    YAG l.
**laser-induced thrombosis**
**laserprobe catheter**
**Lasix**
**Lastac system**
**late**
    l. apical systolic
      murmur
    l. death
    l. deceleration
    l. diastolic murmur
    l. reperfusion
    l. systole
    l. systolic murmur
**lateral**
    l. myocardial infarction
    l. sac
**latex balloon**
*Lathyrus odoratus*
**latissimus dorsi procedure**
*Latrodectus*
**Laurence-Moon-Bardet-Biedl
syndrome**
**Laurence-Moon-Biedl syndrome**
**lavage**
    bronchoalveolar l. (BAL)
**law**
    Bowditch's l.
    Du Bois-Reymond's l.
    Einthoven's l.

    Laplace's l. of heart
    Marey's l.
    Ohm's l.
    Poiseuille's l.
    Sutton's l.
    Torricelli's l.
**LAX**
    long axis
**laxa**
    cutis l.
**layer**
    fascial l.
    half-value l.
    subendocardial l.
**LBBB**
    left bundle branch block
**LCAT**
    lecithin-cholesterol
    acyltransferase
**LCX**
    left circumflex
**LDL**
    low-density lipoprotein
**lead**
    ABC l.'s
    l. apron
    bipolar l.
    CB l.
    CCS endocardial
      pacing l.
    CF l.
    chest l.'s
    CL l.
    cordis l.'s
    CR l.
    direct l.
    Elema l.'s
    endocardial balloon l.
    endocardial cardiac l.
    epicardial l.
    esophageal l.
    indirect l.
    intracardiac l.
    limb l.

Medtronic l.'s
myocardial l.
pacemaker l.'s
permanent cardiac
  pacing l.
permanent pacing l.
l. poisoning
precordial l.'s
semidirect l.'s
standard l.
l. system
telectronic l.'s
temporary pervenous l.
unipolar l.'s
V l.
Vitatron l.'s
**12-lead echocardiography**
**12-lead electrocardiography**
**leading**
l. circle concept
l. circle hypothesis
l. edge
l. edge enhancement
**lead-letter marker**
**leaflet**
anterior l.
aortic valve l.
mitral valve l.
posterior l.
l. thickening
**leakage**
**Lebsche sternal knife**
**lecithin**
**lecithin-cholesterol**
  **acyltransferase (LCAT)**
**ledge**
limbic l.
**left**
l. anterior descending
  artery (LAD)
l. anterior hemiblock
  (LAH)
l. anterior oblique
  (LAO)

l. anterior oblique
  position
l. anterior oblique
  projection
l. aortic angiography
l. atrial angiography
l. atrial appendage
l. atrial dimension
l. atrial emptying index
l. atrial enlargement
l. atrial hypertension
l. atrial myxoma
l. atrial partitioning
l. atrial pressure
l. atrial thrombus
l. atrium
l. axis deviation (LAD)
l. bundle branch block
  (LBBB)
l. circumflex artery
l. coronary artery
l. coronary catheter
l. dominant coronary
  circulation
l. heart
l. heart catheter
l. heart catheterization
l. internal jugular vein
l. internal mammary
  artery (LIMA)
l. lateral projection
l. main coronary artery
l. main coronary artery
  disease
l. main coronary
  stenosis
l. main equivalency
l. main vessel coronary
  stenosis
l. middle hemiblock
l. posterior hemiblock
l. septal hemiblock
l. ventricle (LV)
l. ventricular aneurysm

**left** *(continued)*
l. ventricular angiography
l. ventricular assist device (LVAD)
l. ventricular chamber compliance
l. ventricular diastolic phase index
l. ventricular diastolic pressure
l. ventricular dysfunction
l. ventricular ejection fraction (LVEF)
l. ventricular ejection time (LVET)
l. ventricular end-diastolic pressure (LVEDP)
l. ventricular end-diastolic volume
l. ventricular end-systolic stress
l. ventricular failure
l. ventricular filling pressure
l. ventricular forces
l. ventricular function
l. ventricular hypertrophy (LVH)
l. ventricular inflow tract obstruction
l. ventricular internal dimension
l. ventricular-left atrial crossover dynamics
l. ventricular muscle compliance
l. ventricular myxoma
l. ventricular outflow tract (LVOT)
l. ventricular outflow tract obstruction
l. ventricular outflow tract velocity
l. ventricular output
l. ventricular power
l. ventricular pressure
l. ventricular pressure-volume curve
l. ventricular puncture
l. ventricular-right atrial communication murmur
l. ventricular stress
l. ventricular stroke volume
l. ventricular systolic performance
l. ventricular systolic pressure
l. ventricular tension
l. ventricular volume
l. ventricular wall
l. ventricular wall motion abnormality
l. ventricular wall stress
l. ventriculography
**left circumflex (LCX)**
**left-to-right shunt**
***Legionella***
**Legionnaires' disease**
**Lehman**
L. catheter
L. ventriculography catheter
**leiomyoma**, pl. **leiomyomata**
**leishmaniasis**
**Lenègre's**
L. disease
L. syndrome
**length-active tension curve**
**length-dependent activation**
**length-resting tension relation**
**length-tension relation**
**lens**
sapphire l.
**Lente insulin**

lentigines
lentigines, atrial myxoma, mucocutaneous myxomas, and blue nevi (LAMB)
lentigines, electrocardiographic abnormalities, ocular hypertelovism, pulmonary stenosis, abnormalities of genitalia, retardation of growth, and sensorineural deafness (LEOPARD)
lentiginosis
lentigo, pl. lentigines
lentis
    ectopia l.
LEOPARD
    lentigines, electrocardiographic abnormalities, ocular hypertelovism, pulmonary stenosis, abnormalities of genitalia, retardation of growth, and sensorineural deafness
    LEOPARD syndrome
lepidic cell
leptospirosis
*Leptotrichia buccalis*
Leriche's syndrome
Lescol
lesion
    Bracht-Wachter l.
    branch l.
    coronary artery l.
    de novo l.
    fibromusculoelastic l.
    Janeway l.
    Libman-Sacks l.
    long l.
    monotypic l.
    nonbacterial thrombotic endocardial l.
    restenosis l.
    tandem l.

lethal arrhythmia
leucine
leukemia
leukocyte
    polymorphonuclear l.
leukocytoblastic vasculitis
leukocytoelastic angiitis
leukotriene
level
    blood oxygen l.'s
    multiple shunt l.'s
    reflecting l.
Levine's sign
levocardia malposition
levocardiogram
levodopa
levogram
levoisomerism
Levophed
levo-transposed position
levotransposition
levoversion
Lev's
    L. disease
    L. syndrome
Lewis lines
Libman-Sacks
    L.-S. endocarditis
    L.-S. lesion
    L.-S. syndrome
licorice
lidocaine
lidoflazine
Liebermeister's rule
life
    l. change unit
    l. expectancy
Life Flight helicopter
Lifeline electrode
lift
ligament
    conus l.
    Marshall's l.
    pericardiosternal l.

**ligamentum arteriosum**
**ligation clip**
**ligature**
    Stannius l.
**light**
    laser l.
**lignocaine**
    M l.
**Lillehei-Kaster**
    L.-K. cardiac valve
      prosthesis
    L.-K. pivoting-disc valve
**LIMA**
    left internal mammary
      artery
**limb**
    anacrotic l.
    l. ischemia
    l. lead
**limb-girdle muscular dystrophy**
**limbic ledge**
**limit**
    Nyquist l.
**line**
    arterial l.
    central venous l.
    Conradi's l.
    indwelling l.
    isoelectric l.
    Kerley A l.
    Kerley B l.
    Lewis l.'s
    M l.'s
    Z l.
**linearity**
    amplitude l.
    count-rate l.
**linear phonocardiograph**
**linoleic acid**
**Linx**
    L. extension wire
    L. guide wire extension
    L. wire

*drive*

**lipase**
    diacylglycerol l.
    hepatic l.
    lipoprotein l. (LPL)
**lipid**
    endogenous l.
    exogenous l.
    l. hypothesis
    renomedullary l.
    sarcolemma l.
    l. solubility
**lipid-A**
**lipidosis**, pl. **lipidoses**
**lipocardiac**
**lipodystrophy**
    intestinal l.
**lipofuscinosis**
    neuronal ceroid l.
**lipogenic theory of**
  **atherosclerosis**
**lipoma**
**lipomatous hypertrophy**
**lipoprotein**
    alpha l.
    beta l.
    high-density l. (HDL)
    intermediate-density l.
    l. lipase (LPL)
    low-density l. (LDL)
    pre-beta l.
    triglyceride-rich l.'s
     (TRL)
    very low-density l.
**liposarcoma**
**lisinopril**
**Lissajou loop**
*Listeria monocytogenes*
**list mode**
**lithium**
    l. battery
    l. pacemaker

**lithotripsy**
    extracorporeal shock
      wave l. (ESWL)
    shock wave l.
**Litten's phenomenon**
**Little's disease**
**Litwak mitral valve scissors**
**livedo reticularis**
**liver**
    cardiac l.
    cirrhosis of l.
**l loop**
**load**
    electronic pacemaker l.
    heat l.
**loading**
    relaxation l.
    volume l.
**lobe**
    side l.
**local**
    l. anesthesia
    l. asphyxia
**localization**
    anatomic l.
**localized pericarditis**
**locking**
    l. collar
    l. device
**LOCM**
   low osmolality contrast
    material
**locus**
    genetic l.
**lofexidine**
**Löffler's, Loeffler's**
    L. bacillus
    L. disease
    L. endocarditis
    L. fibroplastic
      endocarditis
    L. syndrome

**logarithmic**
    l. dynamic range
    l. phonocardiograph
**long**
    l. axial oblique view
    l. axis (LAX)
    l. lesion
    l. pulse
    l. Q-T syndrome
**long-acting nitrate**
**long-axis view**
**longitudinal dissociation**
**Loniten**
**loop**
    bulboventricular l.
    d l.
    l. diuretic
    elliptical l.
    guide wire l.
    heart l.
    Henle's l.
    l l.
    Lissajou l.
    memory l.
    P l.
    QRS l.
    T l.
    Uresil radiopaque
      silicone band vessel l.'s
    U-shaped catheter l.
    vector l.
    ventricular pressure-
      volume l.
    video l.
**loose junction**
**Lopid**
**Lopressor**
**Lo-Profile balloon catheter**
**lorazepam**
**lorcainide**
**Lorelco**
**losartin**
**loss of consciousness**
**Lotensin**

**Louis' angle**
**lovastatin**
**low**
    l. fat diet
    l. osmolality contrast
    material (LOCM)
    l. salt diet
    l. salt syndrome
    l. sodium diet
    l. sodium syndrome
**low-density lipoprotein (LDL)**
**Löwenberg's cuff sign**
**lower**
    l. extremity bypass graft
    l. nodal extrasystole
    l. nodal rhythm
**Lown-Ganong-Levine syndrome**
**low-output heart failure**
**low-pressure tamponade**
**Lozol**
**LPL**
  lipoprotein lipase
**lubricity**
**Ludiomil**
**Luer-Lok**
    L.-L. connector
    L.-L. needle
    L.-L. needle tip
**lues**
**luetic**
    l. aortitis
    l. disease
**lumbar sympathectomy**
**Lumelec pacing catheter**
**lumen**
**lumina**
**luminal narrowing**
**lung**
    l. biopsy
    cardiac l.
    l. function
    postperfusion l.
    pump l.
    l. scan

    l. scanning
    shock l.
**lunula, pl. lunulae**
**lupus**
    l. anticoagulant
    l. erythematosus
**Lurselle**
**lusitrophy**
**Lutembacher's**
    L. complex
    L. syndrome
**luxus heart**
**LV**
  left ventricle
**LVAD**
  left ventricular assist device
**LVEDP**
  left ventricular end-diastolic
  pressure
**LVEF**
  left ventricular ejection
  fraction
**LVET**
  left ventricular ejection time
**LVH**
  left ventricular hypertrophy
**LVOT**
  left ventricular outflow tract
**Lyme disease**
**lymphadenopathy**
**lymphangioendothelioma**
**lymphangioma**
**lymphatic**
    l. channel
    obtuse marginal l.
    subclavian l.
**lymphedema**
**lymph node**
**lymphocyte**
**lymphoma**
    B-cell l.
    non-Hodgkin's l.
**lymphomatoid granulomatosis**
**lymphosarcoma**

Lyon hypothesis
lysis time

lysosomal enzyme
lysosome

**mA**
  milliampere
**MacCallum's patch**
**Machado-Guerreiro test**
**machine**
  heart-lung m.
**machinery murmur**
**Mackenzie's polygraph**
**macrocardia**
**macrophage**
**macula,** pl. **maculae**
  m. albida, pl. maculae
    albidae
  m. lactea
  m. tendinea
**Maestro implantable cardiac pacemaker**
**magna**
**magnesium**
  m. sulfate
**magnetic**
  m. moment
  m. record
  m. relaxation time
  m. resonance imaging
    (MRI)
  m. resonance signal
  m. resonance
    spectroscopy
**magnetocardiography**
**magnet pacing interval**
**magnet rate**
**magnification**
**magnitude**
  average pulse m.
  peak m.
**Mahaim fibers**
**malabsorption**
**maladie**
  m. de Roger
**malaria**

**maleate**
  enalapril m.
  ergonovine m.
  nomifensine m.
  timolol m.
  trimipramine m.
**malformation**
  arteriovenous m.
  pulmonary
    arteriovenous m.
    (PAVM)
  Uhl's m.
**malfunction**
  pacemaker m.
**malignancy**
**malignant**
  m. carcinoid syndrome
  m. endocarditis
  m. hypertension
  m. ventricular
    arrhythmia
**malingering**
**Mallory-Weiss syndrome**
**malnutrition**
  alcoholic m.
  protein-calorie m.
**malonylcoenzyme A, malonyl-CoA**
**malposition**
  crisscross heart m.
  dextrocardia m.
  double-outlet left
    ventricle m.
  double-outlet right
    ventricle m.
  ectopia cordis m.
  m. of great arteries
    (MGA)
  levocardia m.
  mesocardia m.
  single ventricle m.
**maltase deficiency**

**malum**
    m. cordis
**mammary**
    m. artery
    m. artery graft
    m. souffle
    m. souffle murmur
**managed care**
**management**
    data base m.
    postprocedural m.
**mandrel**
**maneuver**
    Addison's m.
    cold pressor testing m.
    Ejrup m.
    Heimlich m.
    hemodynamic m.
    Hillis-Müller m.
    hyperventilation m.
    Müller m.
    Valsalva m.
**maneuverability**
**manifest vector**
**manifold**
**manipulation**
    catheter m.
**mannitol**
**manometer**
    Hürthle m.
    m. tipped catheter
**Manoplax**
**Mansfield**
    M. Atri-Pace I catheter
    M. balloon
    M. balloon catheter
    M. bioptome
    M. Valvuloplasty
    Registry
**manual edge detection**
**MAO inhibitor**
**MAP**
    mean arterial pressure

**mapping**
    body surface m.
    bull's eye polar
    coordinate m.
    cardiac m.
    catheter m.
    color-coded flow m.
    electrophysiologic m.
    flow m.
    intraoperative m.
    pace m., pacemapping
    pulsed-wave Doppler m.
    tachycardia pathway m.
    ventricular m.
**maprotiline**
**marantic**
    m. endocarditis
    m. thrombosis
    m. thrombus
**marasmic**
    m. thrombosis
    m. thrombus
**marasmus**
**Marey's law**
**Marfan's**
    M. syndrome
    M. syndrome
    aortography
**marginal**
    m. arteries of
    Drummond
    m. artery
    m. artery of colon
**marginal artery**
    first obtuse m. a.
    (OM-1)
    second obtuse m. a.
    (OM-2)
**marginatum**
    erythema m.
**mark**
    alignment m.
**marker**
    m. catheter

lead-letter m.
vein graft ring m.
**Maroteaux-Lamy syndrome**
**Marshall's**
 M. ligament
 M. oblique vein
 M. vein
**Martorell's syndrome**
**mask**
 ecchymotic m.
**mask-mode**
 m.-m. cardiac imaging
 m.-m. subtraction
**Mason-Likar limb lead modification**
**mass**
 cardiac m.
 intracardiac m.
 myocardial m.
**massage**
 cardiac m.
 carotid sinus m.
 closed-chest cardiac m.
 external cardiac m.
 open-chest cardiac m.
**MAST**
 military anti-shock trousers
**Master's**
 M. test
 M. two-step exercise test
**Masy angioscope**
**matching**
 afterload m.
**material**
 contrast m.
 embolized foreign m.
 Kifa catheter m.
 low osmolality contrast m. (LOCM)
**matrix mode**
**Matsuda titanium surgical instruments**

**Maxilith pacemaker pulse generator**
**maximal velocity ($V_{MAX}$)**
**maximum**
 m. flow rate
 m. negative potential
**Maxzide**
**Mayo hemostat**
**MB fraction**
**McArdle's**
 M. disease
 M. syndrome
**McGoon technique**
**MCV**
 mean corpuscular volume
**MDF**
 myocardial depressant factor
**Meadows' syndrome**
**Meadox**
 M. graft sizer
 M. Teflon felt pledget
**mean**
 m. arterial pressure (MAP)
 m. corpuscular volume (MCV)
 m. diastolic left ventricular pressure
 m. electrical axis
 m. normalized systolic ejection rate
 m. systolic left ventricular pressure
 m. vector
**measurement**
 blood flow m.
 cardiac output m.
 coronary blood flow m.
 Doppler m.
 gas clearance m.
 invasive pressure m.
 physiologic m.
 physiological m.
 PR-AC m.

139

**measurement** *(continued)*
    pressure m.
    thermodilution m.
    venous flow m.
**mechanical**
    m. alternation
    m. valve
    m. ventilation
**mechanics**
    fluid m.
**mechanism**
    m. of action
    Frank-Starling m.
    gating m.
    Starling m.
    steal m.
**mechanocardiography**
**mechanoreflex**
**media**
    arterial m.
**medial tear**
**median**
    m. nerve injury
    m. sternotomy incision
**mediastinum**
**Medical Research Council (MRC)**
**medical therapy**
**Medinvent stent**
**medionecrosis**
    m. of aorta
    m. aortae idiopathica cystica
**Medi-Tech**
    M.-T. balloon catheter
    M.-T. catheter system
    M.-T. guide wire
    M.-T. multipurpose basket
    M.-T. steerable catheter
**Mediterranean anemia**
**medium**
    contrast m.

**Medtronic**
    M. connector
    M. Elite DDDR pacemaker
    M. leads
    M. pacemaker
    M. PCD implantable cardioverter-defibrillator
    M. pulse generator
**Medtronic-Hall (MH)**
    M.-H. valve
**medulla**
    adrenal m.
    m. oblongata
**medullary collecting duct**
**megacardia**
**megaelectron volt (MeV)**
**megaloblastic anemia**
**megalocardia**
**meglumine**
    ioxaglate m.
**meiosis**
**melanoma**
**melioidosis**
**Mellaril**
**membrane**
    alveolar-capillary m., alveolocapillary m.
    cell m.
    m. channel
    cuprophane m.
    Gore-Tex surgical m.
    Henle's elastic m.
    Henle's fenestrated m.
    polyacrylonitrile m.
    m. potential
**membrane-stabilizing activity**
**membranous septum**
**memory**
    cardiac m.
    m. catheter
    m. loop
**mendelian disorder**
**Menghini needle**

*meningitides*
    *Neisseria m.*
meningitis, pl. **meningitides**
meningococcal pericarditis
meningococcemia
meningococcus
menopause
mental
    m. retardation
    m. status
    m. stress
meperidine
    m. hydrochloride
mepivacaine hydrochloride
meralluride
mercaptomerin sodium
Mercuhydrin
mercury (Hg)
    m. poisoning
mercury-195m ($^{195m}$Hg)
Merendino technique
meridional wall stress
merodiastolic
meromyosin
merosystolic
Mersilene suture
mesaortitis
mesarteritis
mesenteric
    m. angiography
    m. arteritis
    m. artery occlusion
    m. bypass graft
    m. ischemia
    m. occlusion
    m. vascular occlusion
mesenteric ischemia
    nonocclusive m. i.
    recurrent m. i.
    transient m. i.
mesenteric vascular occlusion
    inferior m. v. o.
    recurrent m. v. o.

    superior m. v. o.
    venous m. v. o.
mesocardia malposition
mesoderm
    precardiac m.
mesodiastolic
mesophlebitis
mesosystolic
mesothelioma
messenger
    second m.'s
Mestinon
mesylate
    doxazosin m.
    phentolamine m.
MET
    metabolic equivalent
metabolic
    m. acidosis
    m. alkalosis
    m. encephalopathy
    m. equivalent (MET)
    m. parameter
      determination
    m. rate meter
metabolism
    aerobic m.
    anaerobic m.
    glucose m.
    myocardial m.
Metahydrin
metal
    heavy m.
    trace m.
metarteriole
metastasis, pl. **metastases**
    cardiac m.
metastatic
    m. carcinoid syndrome
    m. disease
    m. sarcoma
metazoal myocarditis
Metenix

**meter**
    metabolic rate m.
**methacholine test**
**Methahydrin**
**methanesulfonate**
    phentolamine m.
**methemoglobinemia**
**methicillin**
**methimazole**
**method**
    area-length m.
    atrial extrastimulus m.
    catheter introduction m.
    Douglas bag m.
    dye m.
    dye dilution m.
    Eggleston m.
    Fick m.
    Fick oxygen m.
    Gärtner's m.
    gas clearance m.
    Gräupner's m.
    indocyanine green m.
    King's biopsy m.
    Konno biopsy m.
    Narula m.
    Orsi-Grocco m.
    oxygen step-up m.
    Pachon's m.
    polarographic m.
    sliding scale m.
    Stanford biopsy m.
    Strauss m.
    thermodilution m.
**methotrexate**
**methoxamine hydrochloride**
**methoxyisobutyl isonitrile**
**methyclothiazide**
**methyldopa**
**methylphenidate**
**methylprednisolone**
**methylxanthine**
**methysergide**
**metoclopramide hydrochloride**

**metocurine iodide**
**metolazone**
**metoprolol**
    m. succinate
    m. tartrate
**metrizamide**
**Metroxamine**
**metyrosine**
**Metzenbaum scissors**
**MeV**
    megaelectron volt
**Mevacor**
**mevinolin**
**mexiletine**
    m. hydrochloride
**Mexitil**
**MGA**
    malposition of great arteries
**m gate**
**MH**
    Medtronic-Hall
      MH valve
**MI**
    myocardial infarction
**miconazole**
**microangiopathic anemia**
**microangiopathy**
    thrombotic m.
**microballoon**
    Rand m.
**microbubble**
**micro bulldog clip**
**microcardia**
**microembolism**
**microjoule**
**Microknit patch graft**
**Microlith pacemaker pulse**
  **generator**
**micromanometer**
    m. catheter system
    catheter-tip m. system
**microparticle**
**microsecond pulsed flashlamp**
  **pumped dye laser**

**microsphere**
    radiolabeled m.
**microsphygmy**
**microsphyxia**
**Micross dilatation catheter**
**microvascular clamp**
**micturition syncope**
**Midamor**
**midazolam**
**mid-diastolic murmur**
**midnodal**
    m. extrasystole
    m. rhythm
**midsystolic**
    .m. buckling
    m. click syndrome
    m. murmur
**mifarmonab**
**migraine**
    m. headache
    syncopal m.
    m. syncope
**migrans**
    larva m.
    visceral larva m.
**Mikro-Tip**
    M.-T. catheter
    M.-T. transducer
**Miles vena cava clip**
**miliary embolism**
**MILIS**
    Multicenter Investigation for the Limitation of Infarct Size
**military anti-shock trousers (MAST)**
**milk spot**
**Millar**
    M. catheter

    M. Mikro-Tip catheter
    pressure transducer
    M. transducer
**milliampere (mA)**
**millijoule (mJ)**
**millisecond (msec)**
**mill wheel murmur**
**milrinone**
**mineralocorticoid**
**Minilith pacemaker pulse generator**
**Minipress**
**Minitran**
**Minizide**
**minoxidil**
**minute**
    beats per m. (bpm)
    minute output
**miocardia**
**miosphygmia**
**mirror-image dextrocardia**
**mismatching**
    afterload m.
**mitochondrial function**
**mitochondrion,** pl. **mitochondria**
**mitogen**
**mitoxantrone hydrochloride**
**mitral**
    m. annulus
    m. area
    m. atresia
    m. balloon commissurotomy
    m. balloon valvotomy
    m. buttonhole
    m. click
    m. commissurotomy
    m. facies
    m. gradient
    m. incompetence
    m. insufficiency
    m. murmur
    m. opening snap (MOS)
    m. prolapse

**mitral** *(continued)*
    m. prolapse murmur
    m. prosthesis
    m. regurgitation
    m. regurgitation murmur
    m. restenosis
    m. stenosis
    m. stenosis murmur
    m. tap
    m. valve
    m. valve aneurysm
    m. valve annulus
    m. valve area (MVA)
    m. valve closure index
    m. valve
      echocardiography
    m. valve endocarditis
    m. valve gradient
      (MVG)
    m. valve hypoplasia
    m. valve leaflet
    m. valve prolapse
      (MVP)
    m. valve prolapse
      syndrome
    m. valve replacement
    m. valve valvotomy
    m. valvulitis
    m. valvuloplasty
**mitralis**
    facies m.
**mitral stenosis**
    calcific m.s.
    congenital m.s.
    subvalvular m.s.
**mitral valve**
    cleft m.v.
    flail m.v.
    m.v. prolapse (MVP)
    Starr-Edwards m.v.
    St. Jude m.v.
**mixed**
    m. beat

    m. thrombus
    m. venous blood
**mJ**
    millijoule
**M lignocaine**
**M lines**
**M-mode**
    M.-m. echocardiography
    M.-m. recording
**mobile**
    m. coronary care unit
**Mobin-Uddin**
    M.-U. filter
    M.-U. filter system
    M.-U. vena cava filter
**Mobitz**
    M. atrioventricular block
    M. block
    M. type I
      atrioventricular block
    M. type II
      atrioventricular block
    M. types of
      atrioventricular block
**mode**
    A m.
    fixed rate m.
    gated list m.
    histogram m.
    list m.
    matrix m.
    passive m.
**model**
    Cox proportional
      hazard m.
    Hodgkin-Huxley m.
**Model 40-400 Pruitt-Inahara**
  **shunt**
**moderate hypothermia**
**moderator band**
**modification**
    Mason-Likar limb
      lead m.
    Mullins m.

**modified**
 m. brachial technique
 m. Bruce protocol
**modulus**
 impedance m.
**Moduretic**
**moexipril**
**molsydomine**
**moment**
 magnetic m.
**Mönckeberg's**
 M. arteriosclerosis
 M. degeneration
**Mondor's**
 M. disease
 M. syndrome
**Monge's disease**
**mongolism**
*moniliformis*
 *Streptobacillus m.*
**Monit**
**monitor**
 cardiac m.
 Criticare
  ETCO2/SpO2 m.
 electronic fetal m.
 Holter m.
 Nellcor Nl000
  ETCO2/SpO2 m.
 video m.
**monitoring**
 ambulatory m.
 physiological m.
**monoamine**
 m. oxidase
 m. oxidase inhibitor
  (MAO inhibitor)
**monocardiogram**
**Mono-Cedocard**
**monoclonal**
 m. antibody
 m. hypothesis
 m. theory of
  atherogenesis

**monocrotaline**
**monocrotic pulse**
**monocrotism**
**monocyte**
*monocytogenes*
 *Listeria m.*
**monofoil catheter**
**Monoker**
**monometer-tipped catheter**
**mononitrate**
 isosorbide m.
**mononucleosis**
 infectious m.
**monophasic complex**
**monophosphate**
 adenosine m. (AMP)
 cyclic adenosine m.
  (cAMP)
 guanosine m. (GMP)
**monopolar temporary electrode**
**Monopril**
**monotypic lesion**
**monoxide**
 carbon m.
*Moraxella*
**morbidity**
**Moretz clip**
**Morgagni-Adams-Stokes**
 **syndrome**
**Morgagni's disease**
**moribund**
**moricizine**
**morphine**
**morphologic**
**morphology**
**Morquio's syndrome**
**mortality**
 operative m.
 m. rate
**MOS**
 mitral opening snap
**mosquito**
 m. clamp
 m. hemostat

**Mosso's sphygmomanometer**
**motion**
    atrioventricular
      junction m.
    diastolic m.
    m. display echo
    interventricular
      septal m.
    precordial m.
    systolic m.
    ventricular wall m.
    wall m.
**Motrin**
**mountain sickness**
**mousetail pulse**
**mouth-to-mouth**
    m.-t.-m. resuscitation
    m.-t.-m. ventilation
**movable**
    m. core straight safety
      wire guide
    m. heart
    m. pulse
**movement**
    m. disorder
    precordial m.
**moxalactam**
**moyamoya disease**
**M protein**
**M-protein serotype**
**MRC**
    Medical Research Council
**MRFIT**
    Multiple-Risk Factor
    Intervention Trial
**MRI**
    magnetic resonance imaging
**MRM-2**
**msec**
    millisecond
**mucocutaneous lymph node**
  **syndrome**
**mucoid medial degeneration**
**mucolipidosis,** pl. **mucolipidoses**

**mucopolysaccharide**
    acid m. (AMP)
**mucopolysaccharidosis,**
  pl. **mucopolysaccharidoses**
*Mucor*
**mucormycosis**
**MUGA**
    multiple gated acquisition
    MUGA scan
**Müller's**
    M. experiment
    M. maneuver
    M. sign
**Müller vena caval clamp**
**Mullins**
    M. catheter
    M. dilator
    M. modification
    M. sheath
    M. sheath/dilator
    M. sheath system
    M. transseptal
      catheterization sheath
**Multicenter Investigation for**
  **the Limitation of Infarct**
  **Size (MILIS)**
**Multicor cardiac pacemaker**
**multi-element linear array**
**multifocal tachycardia**
**multiforme**
    erythema m.
**multiform premature**
  **ventricular complex**
**multilayer design catheter**
**Multilith pacemaker**
**multiple**
    m. balloon valvuloplasty
    m. embolism
    m. gated acquisition
    (MUGA)
    m. lentigines syndrome
    m. lipoprotein-type
    hyperlipidemia
    m. regression

m. sclerosis
m. shunt levels
m. system atrophy
**Multiple-Risk Factor Intervention Trial (MRFIT)**
**multipurpose**
m. catheter
m. technique
**multisensor catheter**
**multivalvular**
m. disease
m. disease murmur
**multivessel**
m. coronary artery obstruction
m. disease
*multocida*
*Pasteurella m.*
**mumps**
**mural**
m. aneurysm
m. endocarditis
m. thrombosis
m. thrombus
**murmur**
accidental m.
anemic m.
aortic m.
aortic-left ventricular tunnel m.
aortic-mitral combined disease m.
aortic regurgitation m.
aortic stenosis m.
apical mid-diastolic heart m.
apical systolic heart m.
arterial m.
atriosystolic m.
atrioventricular flow rumbling m.
Austin Flint m.
bellows m.
blowing m.

brain m.
bronchial collateral artery m.
Cabot-Locke m.
carcinoid m.
cardiac m.
cardiopulmonary m.
cardiorespiratory m.
Carey Coombs m.
carotid artery m.
Cole-Cecil m.
continuous m.
continuous heart m.
Coombs m.
crescendo m.
crescendo-decrescendo m.
Cruveilhier-Baumgarten m.
decrescendo m.
diamond-shaped m.
diastolic m.
Duroziez' m.
dynamic m.
early diastolic m.
early-peaking systolic m.
early systolic m.
ejection m.
endocardial m.
exocardial m.
extracardiac m.
Flint's m.
Fräntzel's m.
friction m.
functional m.
Gibson m.
Graham Steell's m.
heart m.
hemic m.
Hodgkin-Key m.
holosystolic m.
hourglass m.
innocent m.
innocent m. of elderly
inorganic m.

**murmur** *(continued)*
    late apical systolic m.
    late diastolic m.
    late systolic m.
    left ventricular-right
      atrial
      communication m.
    machinery m.
    mammary souffle m.
    mid-diastolic m.
    midsystolic m.
    mill wheel m.
    mitral m.
    mitral prolapse m.
    mitral regurgitation m.
    mitral stenosis m.
    multivalvular disease m.
    muscular m.
    musical m.
    nun's m.
    obstructive m.
    organic m.
    pansystolic m.
    patent ductus
      arteriosus m.
    pathologic m.
    pericardial m.
    pleuropericardial m.
    presystolic m.
    primary pulmonary
      hypertension m.
    pulmonary m.,
      pulmonic m.
    regurgitant m.
    Roger's m.
    seagull m.
    seesaw m.
    Steell's m.
    stenosal m.
    Still's m.
    systolic m.
    systolic regurgitant m.
    to-and-fro m.
    tricuspid m.

    vascular m.
    venous m.
    ventricular septal
      defect m.
    water wheel m.
**muscarinic receptor**
**muscle**
    m. bridge
    cardiac m.
    papillary m.
    m. relaxant
    skeletal m.
    m. stiffness
    venous smooth m.
**muscular**
    m. dystrophy
    m. incompetence
    m. murmur
    m. subaortic stenosis
**musculoskeletal pain**
**musical murmur**
**Musset's sign**
**Mustard**
    M. interatrial baffle
    M. operation
    M. procedure
**mutant allele**
**mutation**
**muzolimine**
**MVA**
    mitral valve area
**MVE-50 implantable**
   **myocardial electrode**
**MVG**
    mitral valve gradient
**MVP**
    mitral valve prolapse
**myasthenia**
    m. cordis
    m. gravis
***Mycobacterium***
    *M. avium*
    *M. bovis*
    *M. chelonei*

M. *fortuitum*
M. *gordonae*
M. *intracellulare*
M. *tuberculosis*
**Mycoplasma pneumoniae**
**Mycoscint**
**mycotic**
 m. aneurysm
 m. aortic aneurysm
 m. aortography
**mydriatic**
**myeloma**
**Mylar catheter**
**myocardial**
 m. abscess
 m. anoxia
 m. bridge
 m. bridging
 m. clamp
 m. concussion
 m. contractility
 m. contusion
 m. depolarization
 m. depressant factor (MDF)
 m. depression
 m. disease
 m. edema
 m. failure
 m. fiber shortening
 m. function
 m. hibernation
 m. hypertrophy
 m. imaging
 m. infarction (MI)
 m. infarction in H-form
 m. injury
 m. insufficiency
 m. ischemia
 m. ischemic syndrome
 m. lead
 m. mass
 m. metabolism

 m. muscle creatine kinase isozyme (CK-MB)
 m. necrosis
 m. oxygen consumption
 m. oxygen demand
 m. oxygen supply
 m. oxygen uptake
 m. perforation
 m. perfusion
 m. perfusion imaging
 m. perfusion scintigraphy
 m. perfusion study
 m. rigor mortis
 m. rupture
 m. stiffness
 m. stunning
 m. tension
 m. tissue
 m. viability
**myocardial infarction (MI)**
 acute m. i. (AMI)
 atrial m. i.
 completed m. i.
 complicated m. i.
 silent m. i.
 subendocardial m. i.
 transmural m. i.
**myocardiograph**
**myocardiopathy**
**myocardiorraphy**
**myocarditis**
 acute isolated m.
 bacterial m.
 clostridial m.
 coxsackievirus m.
 echovirus m.
 Fiedler's m.
 fragmentation m.
 giant cell m.
 helminthic m.
 hypersensitivity m.
 indurative m.

**myocarditis** *(continued)*
    metazoal m.
    parenchymatous m.
    protozoal m.
    rheumatic m.
    rheumatoid m.
    rickettsial m.
    spirochetal m.
    syphilitic m.
    tuberculoid m.
    viral m.
**myocardium**
    hibernating m.
    ischemic m.
    stunned m.
**myocardosis**
**myocyte**
    m. necrosis
**myocytolysis**
    coagulative m.
    m. of heart
**myoendocarditis**
**myofascial**
**myofibril**
**myofibrillar**
**myofibroblast**
**myofibrosis**
    m. cordis
**myofilament**
**myogenic theory**
**myoglobin**
**myolysis**
    cardiotoxic m.
**myopathia cordis**
**myopathy**
    centronuclear m.

    myotubular m.
    nemaline m.
**myopericarditis**
**Myoscint**
**myosin**
    cardiac m.
**myosin-specific antibody**
**myositis**
**myotomy-myectomy-septal
  resection**
**myotonia**
    m. congenita
**myotonic**
    m. dystrophy
    m. muscular dystrophy
**myotubular myopathy**
**Myowire**
    M. cardiac electrode
    M. II cardiac electrode
**myurous**
**myxoma,** pl. **myxomata**
    atrial m.
    infected m.
    left atrial m.
    left ventricular m.
    right atrial m.
    right ventricular m.
    m. tumor
    ventricular m.
**myxomatous**
    m. degeneration
    m. proliferation
    m. pulmonary embolism

**NAD**
nicotinamide adenine dinucleotide
**nadolol**
**nafazatrom**
**nafcillin**
**nail pulse**
**nalbuphine hydrochloride**
**naloxone hydrochloride**
**NAME**
nevi, atrial myxoma, myxoid neurofibromas, and ephelides
NAME syndrome
**Namic**
N. angiographic syringe
N. catheter
**N-13 ammonia**
**Naqua**
**Narcan**
**narcotic**
**narrowing**
atherosclerotic n.
luminal n.
**Narula method**
**National Heart, Lung and Blood Institute (NHLBI)**
**National Institutes of Health (NIH)**
**native coarctation**
**Natrilix**
**natriuresis**
**natriuretic**
n. hormone
n. peptide
**natural frequency**
**Naturetin**
**Naughton**
N. protocol
N. treadmill protocol

**Nauheim**
N. bath
N. treatment
**Navidrex**
**N cell**
**Nd:YAG laser**
neodymium:yttrium-aluminum-garnet laser
**near field**
**near-gain**
**nebivolol**
**necrobiosis**
n. diabeticorum
n. lipoidica diabeticorum
**necropsy**
**necrosis**, pl. **necroses**
coagulation n.
contraction band n.
cystic medial n.
n. factor
myocardial n.
myocyte n.
renal cortical n.
tissue n.
tubular n.
**necrotizing**
n. angiitis
n. arteriolitis
n. vasculitis
**needle**
argon n.
arterial n.
Brockenbrough n.
Brockenbrough curved n.
Cournand n.
eyeless n.
Fergie n.
Ferguson n.
front wall n.
n. holder
Luer-Lok n.

**needle** *(continued)*
    Menghini n.
    Potts n.
    Potts-Cournand n.
    Rashkind septostomy n.
    Riley n.
    Ross n.
    Seldinger n.
    standard n.
    thin-walled n.
**negative**
    n. chronotropism
    n. contrast
    n. pressure
**negligence**
*Neisseria*
    *N. meningitides*
**Nellcor**
    N. N2500 ETCO2
    multigas analyzer
    N. Nl000 ETCO2/SpO2
    monitor
    N. N200 pulse oximeter
**nemaline myopathy**
**Nembutal**
**neodymium:yttrium-aluminum-garnet laser (Nd:YAG laser, Nd:YAG laser)**
*neoformans*
    *Cryptococcus n.*
**neomycin**
    n. sulfate
**neonatal internal jugular puncture kit**
**neonate**
**neoplasia**
**neoplasm**
**neoplastic**
    n. disease
    n. pericarditis
**neostrophingic**
**neovascularization**

**Nephril**
**nephritis**, pl. **nephritides**
    familial n.
**nephrogram**
**nephron**
**nephropathic cardiomyopathy**
**nephropathy**
    analgesic n.
    diabetic n.
    hyperuricemic n.
**nephrosclerosis**
**nephrotic syndrome**
**nephrotoxicity**
**Nernst equation**
**nerve**
    carotid sinus n.
    hypoglossal n.
    laryngeal n.
    phrenic n.
    sensory n.
    thoracic n.
    vagus n.
**nervosa**
    anorexia n.
**nervous system**
**Nestor-3**
**Nestor guiding catheter**
**network**
    Chiari n.
**neuralgia**
    glossopharyngeal n.
**neuritis**
    optic n.
**neuroblastoma**
**neurocardiac**
**neurocirculatory asthenia**
**neuroendocrine theory**
**neurofibroma**
**neurofibromatosis**
**neurogenic**
    n. pulmonary edema
    n. theory
**neuroleptic**

neurologic
  n. examination
  n. status
neurological disorder
neuromuscular
  n. disease
  n. disorder
neuromyopathic disorder
neuronal ceroid lipofuscinosis
neuropathy
neuropeptide Y
neurosis, pl. neuroses
  anxiety n.
  cardiac n.
neuroticism
neurotoxic effect
neurotransmitter substance
neuroxanthoendothelioma
neutropenia
nevi, atrial myxoma, myxoid
  neurofibromas, and ephelides
  (NAME)
Newton guide wire
New York Heart Association
  (NYHA)
New York Heart Association
  classification
NHLBI
  National Heart, Lung and
  Blood Institute
NH region
niacin
nicardipine
nickel
nickel-cadmium battery
nicofuranose
Nicoladoni-Branham's sign
nicorandil
nicotinamide adenine
  dinucleotide (NAD)
nicotinic acid
Niemann-Pick disease
nifedipine
  n. enzyme immunoassay

Niglycon
NIH
  National Institutes of Health
  NIH catheter
  NIH marking catheter
Niko-Fix
nimodipine
Nimotop
Niong
Nipride
nisoldipine
Nitinol
nitrate
  long-acting n.
nitrendipine
nitrite
  amyl n.
  sodium n.
Nitro-bid
Nitrocap
Nitrocels
Nitrocine
Nitro-Dial
Nitrodisc
Nitro-Dur patch
Nitrodyl
Nitrodyl-B
Nitrogard
nitrogen
nitrogen-13 ammonia
nitroglycerin transdermal patch
nitroglycerol
Nitroglyn
Nitrol
Nitrolin
Nitrolingual
Nitromed
Nitronet
Nitrong
Nitropress
nitroprusside
  n. infusion
  sodium n.
Nitrospan

Nitrostat
Nitro TD
Nitrotym
Nitrotym-Plus
nitrous oxide
Nitrovas
NL3 guider
*Nocardia israelii*
nocturia
nocturnal dyspnea
nodal
    n. arrhythmia
    n. bigeminy
    n. bradycardia
    n. escape
    n. extrasystole
    n. premature contraction
    n. rhythm
    n. tachycardia
    n. tissue
node
    atrioventricular n.
    (AVN)
    lymph n.
    Osler n.
    sinus n., sinoatrial n.
    (SN)
nodosa
    arteritis n.
    periarteritis n.
    polyarteritis n.
nodoventricular tract
nodular sclerosis
nodule
    Albini's n.
    Arantius' n.
    Aschoff n.
    calcified n.
    subcutaneous n.
nodus
    n. atrioventriculosis
    n. sinuatrialis
    n. sinuatrialis echo
nomifensine maleate

nomogram
nonacute total occlusion
nonbacterial
    n. thrombotic
    endocardial lesion
    n. thrombotic
    endocarditis
    n. verrucous
    endocarditis
noncardiac
    n. angiography
    n. surgery
    n. syncope
nondisjunction
nonexertional angina
nonflotation catheter
non flow-directed catheter
nonglycoside inotropic agent
non-Hodgkin's lymphoma
noninvasive
    n. assessment
    n. evaluation
    n. testing
nonionic
nonocclusive mesenteric
    ischemia
nonoperative closure
nonparoxysmal
    n. atrioventricular
    junctional tachycardia
    n. junctional tachycardia
    n. tachycardia
nonpenetrating rupture
nonphasic sinus arrhythmia
non-Q-wave myocardial
    infarction
nonselective coronary
    angiography
nonsteroidal antiinflammatory
    agent
nonthrombogenic
nontransmural myocardial
    infarction (NTMI)
Noonan's syndrome

NoProfile balloon
Norcuron
no-reflow phenomenon
norepinephrine
norethindrone
normal
    n. axis
    n. intravascular pressure
Normodyne
Normotensin
normothermic cardioplegia
Normozide
Norpace
Norpace CR
Norpramin
Norton flow-directed Swan-
  Ganz thermodilution catheter
nortriptyline
    n. hydrochloride
Norvase
Norwood's operation
notch
    anacrotic n.
    aortic n.
    dicrotic n.
notching
Novametrix
    N. ETCO2 multigas
    analyzer
    N. pulse oximeter

Novantrone
Novoste catheter
NPH insulin
N region
NS echo
NTMI
    nontransmural myocardial
    infarction
nuclear
    n. magnetic resonance
    imaging
    n. pacemaker
    n. probe
    n. study
nucleus, pl. nuclei
number
    Reynold's n.
    Strouhal's n.
nun's murmur
Nurolon suture
nutrition
Nyboer esophageal electrode
Nycore-pigtail catheter
NYHA
    New York Heart Association
Nyomin
Nyquist limit

**obesity**
**obesity-hypoventilation**
  **syndrome**
**oblique**
    left anterior o. (LAO)
    right anterior o. (RAO)
    o. sinus
**obliterans**
    arteriosclerosis o.
    arteritis o.
    thromboangiitis o.
**obliterative cardiomyopathy**
**oblongata**
    medulla o.
**obstruction**
    aortic o.
    coronary artery o.
    infundibular o.
    left ventricular inflow
      tract o.
    left ventricular outflow
      tract o.
    multivessel coronary
      artery o.
    outflow tract o.
    pulmonary vascular o.
    right ventricular o.
    right ventricular
      outflow o.
    subpulmonary o.
    subvalvular o.
    vena caval o.
    ventricular inflow
      tract o.
    ventricular outflow
      tract o.
**obstructive**
    o. hypertrophic
      cardiomyopathy
    o. lung disease
    o. murmur

    o. shock
    o. sleep apnea (OSA)
    o. thrombus
**obturating embolism**
**obturator**
    Fitch o.
**obtuse marginal lymphatic**
**occluder**
    air clamp inflatable
      vessel o.
    Brockenbrough curved-
      tip o.
    catheter tip o.
    Crile tip o.
    double disc o.
    Hunter detachable
      balloon o.
    tilting-disk o.
    tip o.
**occlusion**
    angioplasty-related
      vessel o.
    axillary artery o.
    axillary vein o.
    balloon o.
    branch vessel o.
    coronary o.
    coronary artery o.
    femoral artery o.
    femoral vein o.
    iliac artery o.
    inferior vena cava o.
    intermittent coronary
      sinus o.
    mesenteric o.
    mesenteric artery o.
    mesenteric vascular o.
    nonacute total o.
**occlusive**
    o. disease
    o. thromboaortopathy

**occult**
    o. pericardial
      constriction
    o. pericarditis
**ochrometer**
**ochronosis**
**ocular larva migrans**
**oculocardiac reflex**
**oculomucocutaneous syndrome**
**oculoplethysmography**
**oculopneumoplethysmography**
*odoratus*
    *Lathyrus o.*
**odynophagia**
**Ohmeda**
    O. ETCO2 multigas
      analyzer
    O. pulse oximeter
**Ohm's law**
**oil**
    canola o.
    o. embolism
    fish o.
**OKT3 antibody**
**Olbert balloon**
**oligemia**
**oligemic shock**
**olighemia**
**oliguria**
**olivopontocerebellar atrophy**
**Olympus bioptome**
**OM-1**
    first obtuse marginal artery
**OM-2**
    second obtuse marginal
      artery
**omega-3 unsaturated fatty acid**
**Omnicarbon valve**
**Omnicor pacemaker**
**Omnipaque**
**Omniscience**
    O. cardiac valve
      prosthesis
    O. valve

**omphalitis**
**omphalocele**
**omphalomesenteric vein**
**oncotic pressure**
**onychograph**
**opacification**
**opacify**
**opacity**
    vitreous o.
**open-chest cardiac massage**
**open heart surgery**
**opening snap**
**operation**
    arterial switch o.
    Blalock-Hanlon o.
    Blalock-Taussig o.
    Glenn's o.
    Hunter's o.
    Konno o.
    Mustard o.
    Norwood's o.
    Potts' o.
    Rastan o.
    Senning o.
    switch o.
    talc o.
    Trendelenburg's o.
    Waterston's o.
**operative mortality**
**ophthalmoplegia**
**ophthalmotonometry**
**opiate**
**opioid**
**optic**
    o. atrophy
    o. disk
    o. neuritis
**optical fiber catheter**
**Opticath oximeter catheter**
**Optiray contrast**
**oral**
    o. anticoagulant therapy
    o. contraceptive

*oralis*
>*Bacteroides o.*

Oretic
Oreticyl
Oreticyl Forte
organic murmur
orifice
>flow across o.

origin
>anomalous o.

Orsi-Grocco method
orthoarteriotony
orthodromic tachycardia
orthogonal
>o. lead system
>o. plane

orthopercussion
orthopnea
orthostatic
>o. hypertension
>o. hypopiesis
>o. hypotension
>o. syncope

orthotopic cardiac
  transplantation
OSA
>obstructive sleep apnea

Osborne wave
oscillatory afterpotential
oscillometer
oscilloscope
Osler node
Osler's
>O. sign
>O. triad

Osler-Weber-Rendu syndrome
Osmitrol
osmolality
osmometer
osmotic
>o. diuretic
>o. pressure

ossification
>pulmonary o.

osteoarthritis
osteoarthropathy
>hypertrophic
>pulmonary o.

osteogenesis imperfecta
osteosarcoma
ostium, pl. ostia
>coronary o.
>persistent o. primum
>o. primum
>o. primum defect
>o. secundum
>o. secundum defect

Ostwald viscosimeter
ototoxicity
ouabain
outflow
>o. tract
>o. tract obstruction

out-of-hospital cardiac arrest
outpatient
>o. catheterization
>o. procedure

output
>cardiac o.
>Fick cardiac o.
>left ventricular o.
>minute o.
>pacemaker o.
>stroke o.
>thermodilution o.
>thermodilution
>  cardiac o.

ovale
>foramen o.
>patent foramen o.

oval foramen
ovalis
>annulus o.
>fossa o.

overdilation
overdrive
>o. pacing
>o. suppression

**overflow wave**
**overload**
 diastolic o.
 pressure o.
 volume o.
**overreactivity**
 physiological o.
**overriding aorta**
**oversensing**
 o. pacemaker
**oversewing**
**oversight review**
**Owens**
 O. balloon
 O. balloon catheter
 O. catheter
 O. Lo-Profile dilatation
  catheter
**oxacillin**
**oxalate**
 calcium o.
**oxalosis**
**oxandralone**
**oxazepam**
**oxidase**
 monoamine o.
**oxidative phosphorylation**
**oxide**
 nitrous o.
**oximeter**
 Criticare pulse o.
 ear o.

 Nellcor N200 pulse o.
 Novametrix pulse o.
 Ohmeda pulse o.
 pulse o.
 SpaceLabs pulse o.
**oximetry**
 reflectance o.
 spectrophotometric o.
**oxprenolol**
**oxygen**
 blood o. levels
 o. carrying capacity
 o. consumption
 o. consumption index
 o. content
 o. inhalation
 o. paradox
 o. radical
 o. saturation
 o. step-up method
 o. tension
 o. therapy
 o. uptake
**oxygen-15**
**oxygenation**
**oxygenator**
 extracorporeal
  membrane o.
 extracorporeal pump o.
 pump o.
**oxyphenbutazone P$_2$**
**oxysterol inhibitor**

# P

**PA**
  pulmonary artery
**Pa**
  pulmonary arterial pressure
**PAC**
  premature atrial contraction
**Paceart complete pacemaker patient testing system**
**paced rhythm**
**pacemaker**
  Accufix p.
  Acculith p.
  Activitrax p.
  activity-sensing p.
  antitachycardia p. (ATP)
  artificial p.
  Astra p.
  atrial asynchronous p.
  atrial demand p.
  atrial synchronous p.
  atrial synchronous
    ventricular inhibited p.
  Atricor p.
  atrioventricular
    sequential p.
  automatic p.
  Axios 04 p.
  Biotronik p.
  bipolar p.
  p. catheter
  Chardack p.
  Chronocor p.
  Chronos 04 p.
  committed mode p.
  Coratomic p.
  Cordis p.
  Cosmos p.
  Cyberlith p.
  demand p.
  dual chamber p.
  dual demand p.
  ECT p.

  ectopic p.
  electric cardiac p.
  p. electrodes
  Elite p.
  Encor p.
  external p.
  p. failure
  fixed-rate p.
  fully automatic p.
  Galaxy p.
  Gen2 p.
  Hancock bipolar
    balloon p.
  p. impedance
  p. leads
  lithium p.
  Maestro implantable
    cardiac p.
  p. malfunction
  Medtronic p.
  Medtronic Elite
    DDDR p.
  Multicor cardiac p.
  Multilith p.
  nuclear p.
  Omnicor p.
  p. output
  oversensing p.
  Paragon p.
  Paragon II p.
  pervenous p.
  Phoenix p.
  p. pocket
  Poly Flex p.
  Programalith p.
  programmable p.
  Pulsar NI
    implantable p.
  Reflex p.
  Relay p.
  p. sensitivity
  Sensolog III p.

**pacemaker** *(continued)*
    shifting p.
    Siemens-Elema p.
    Solus p.
    Stanicor p.
    subsidiary atrial p.
    Symbios p.
    Synchrony p.
    Synchrony I p.
    Synchrony II p.
    universal p.
    Ventak AICD p.
    ventricular
      asynchronous p.
    ventricular demand p.
    Vista p.
    wandering p.
**pacemapping**
**pace mapping**
**Pacewedge dual-pressure**
  **bipolar pacing catheter**
**Pachon's**
    P. method
    P. test
**pacing**
    AAI p.
    AAIR p.
    AAI-RR p.
    AAT p.
    AOO p.
    asynchronous p.
    atrial p.
    p. catheter
    DDD p.
    DDDR p.
    DDI p.
    dual-chamber p.
    DVI p.
    p. hysteresis
    incremental atrial p.
    inhibited p.
    intracardiac p.
    overdrive p.
    permanent p.

    rapid atrial p.
    rate responsive p.
    p. system analyzer
    temporary p.
    triggered p.
    VAT p.
    VDD p.
    ventricular p.
    VOO p.
    VVI p.
    VVIR p.
    VVI-RR p.
    VVT p.
**P-A conduction time**
**paddle**
    electrode p.
*Paecilomyces*
**Paget's**
    P. disease
    P. disease of bone
**Paget-von Schrötter syndrome**
**pain**
    atypical chest p.
    chest p.
    functional p.
    musculoskeletal p.
    pleuritic chest p.
    psychogenic p.
    pulmonary p.
    rest p.
**P-A interval**
**paired**
    p. beat
    p. electrical stimulation
**palate**
**pale**
    p. hypertension
    p. thrombus
**palliation**
**palliative**
    p. surgery
*pallidum*
    *Treponema p.*
**pallor**

**palmar**
>p. arch
>p. xanthoma

**palmare**
>xanthoma striatum p.

**palmi**
**palmic**
**palmitic acid**
**palmitoylcarnitine**
**palmodic**
**palmoscopy**
**palmus**, pl. **palmi**
**palpation**
>bimanual precordial p.

**palpitatio cordis**
**palpitations**
**Pamelor**
**pancarditis**
**panconduction defect**
**pancreas**
**pancreatitis**
**pancuronium bromide**
**pang**
>breast p.

**panic disorder**
**panniculitis**
**panning**
**panophthalmitis**
**pansystolic**
>p. murmur

**pantaloon embolism**
**pantothenate synthetase**
**pantyhose**
>Glattelast
>compression p.

**Panwarfin**
**panzerherz**
**papaverine**
**papilla**
>Bergmeister's p.

**papillary**
>p. fibroelastoma
>p. muscle
>p. muscle abscess

>p. muscle dysfunction
>p. muscle syndrome
>p. tumor

**papilledema**
**papillitis**
**papillotome**
>Wilson-Cook p.

**papulosis**
>atrophic p.

**para-aminosalicylic acid (PAS, PASA)**
**paracentesis**
>p. cordis
>p. pericardii
>p. thoracis

**paracetamol sensitivity**
**parachute**
>p. deformity
>p. mitral valve
>p. valve

**paradox**
>calcium p.
>p. image
>oxygen p.

**paradoxical**
>p. embolism
>p. embolization
>p. embolus
>p. pulse
>p. split of $S_2$

**paradoxus**
>p. parvus et tardus
>pulsus p.

**paraganglioma**
**Paragon**
>P. II pacemaker
>P. pacemaker

**paralysis**
>ischemic p.
>periodic p.
>tick p.
>vasomotor p.

**paramagnetic substance**
**paramedian**

163

paramedic
parameters
  systemic
    hemodynamic p.
parametric image
pararrhythmia
parasternal
  p. examination
  p. view
parasympathetic
  p. function
  p. nervous system
  p. system
parasystole
parasystolic beat
parathyroid
  p. gland
  p. hormone
paravalvular
parchment heart
parenchymatous myocarditis
parietal
  p. pericardiectomy
  p. thrombus
parieto-occipital artery
park blade septostomy
  catheter
Parlodel
paroxysmal
  p. atrial fibrillation
  p. atrial tachycardia
    (PAT)
  p. junctional tachycardia
  p. nocturnal dyspnea
    (PND)
  p. nodal tachycardia
  p. reentrant
    supraventricular
    tachycardia
  p. supraventricular
    tachycardia
  p. tachycardia
Parsonnet
  P. coronary probe

P. pulse generator
  pouch
partial
  p. occlusion inferior
    vena cava clip
  p. thromboplastin time
    (PTT)
partitioning
  left atrial p.
parvus
  p. alternans
  p. et tardus pulse
  pulsus p.
PAS
  para-aminosalicylic acid
PASA
  para-aminosalicylic acid
passive
  p. clot
  p. congestion
  p. hyperemia
  p. interval
  p. mode
*Pasteurella multocida*
PAT
  paroxysmal atrial
    tachycardia
patch
  Dacron p.
  Dacron intracardiac p.
  Gore-Tex
    cardiovascular p.
  Ionescu-Shiley
    pericardial p.
  MacCallum's p.
  Nitro-Dur p.
  nitroglycerin
    transdermal p.
  polypropylene
    intracardiac p.
  soldier's p.'s
  Teflon intracardiac p.
  transdermal p.

**patency**
  catheter p.
  probe p.
**patent**
  p. ductus arteriosus (PDA)
  p. ductus arteriosus murmur
  p. ductus arteriosus umbrella
  p. foramen ovale
**pathogenesis**
**pathologic murmur**
**pathology**
  coexistent p.
**pathway**
  accessory p.
  conduction p.
  internodal p.'s
  scavenger cell p.
  shunt p.
**patient**
  asymptomatic p.
  p. compliance
  contrast allergic p.
  high-risk p.
  p. transport
**pattern**
  ballerina-foot p.
  contraction p.
  hourglass p.
  intraventricular conduction p.
  juvenile p.
**pause**
  compensatory p.
  postextrasystolic p.
  preautomatic p.
  sinus p.
**Pavlov's reflex**
**PAVM**
  pulmonary arteriovenous malformation
**Pavulon**

**PAWP**
  pulmonary artery wedge pressure
**P cell**
**P-congenitale**
**PDA**
  patent ductus arteriosus
  posterior descending artery
  PDA umbrella
**P-dextrocardiale**
**PDT guide wire**
**PE-60-I-2 implantable pronged unipolar electrode**
**PE-60-K-10 implantable unipolar endocardial electrode**
**PE-60-KB implantable unipolar endocardial electrode**
**PE-85-I-2 implantable pronged unipolar electrode**
**PE-85-K-10 implantable unipolar endocardial electrode**
**PE-85-KB implantable unipolar endocardial electrode**
**PE-85-KS-10 implantable unipolar endocardial electrode**
**peak**
  p. diastolic filling rate
  p. filling rate (PFR)
  p. incidence
  p. magnitude
  p. systolic aortic pressure (PSAP)
  p. systolic gradient (PSG)
  p. systolic gradient pressure
  p. transaortic valve gradient (AVG)
  p. twitch force

**pectoris**
   angina p.
**pectus**
   p. carinatum
   p. excavatum
**pedal pulse**
**pediatric**
   p. cardiomyopathy
   p. hypertension
   p. pigtail catheter
**Pedoff continuous wave transducer**
**Peel-Away introducer set**
**PEEP**
   positive end-expiratory pressure
**peer review**
**pellagra**
**penbutolol**
**pendulous heart**
**pendulum rhythm**
**penetrating**
   p. injury
   p. rupture
**penetration**
**penicillin**
   benzathine benzyl p.
**penicillin G**
*Penicillium*
**Penn State heart**
**pentaerythritol tetranitrate**
**pentalogy**
   Cantrell's p.
   p. of Fallot, Fallot's p.
**pentazocine**
**pentobarbital**
**Pentothal**
**pentoxifylline**
**PEP**
   preejection period
**peptic**
   p. esophagitis
   p. ulcer

**peptide**
   atrial natriuretic p.
   natriuretic p.
**perceived exertion**
**percussion wave**
**percutaneous**
   p. approach
   p. balloon angioplasty
   p. balloon angioplasty of coarctation
   p. balloon aortic valvuloplasty
   p. balloon pulmonic valvuloplasty
   p. balloon valvotomy
   p. balloon valvuloplasty
   p. brachial sheath
   p. catheter insertion
   p. catheter introducer kit
   p. mitral balloon valvotomy
   p. mitral balloon valvuloplasty (PMV)
   p. mitral valvotomy
   p. rotational thrombectomy (PRT)
   p. rotational thrombectomy catheter
   p. technique
   p. transluminal angioplasty
   p. transluminal balloon valvuloplasty
   p. transluminal coronary angioplasty (PTCA)
   p. tunnel
**Perez' sign**
**perforation**
   cardiac p.
   guide wire p.
   myocardial p.
   septal p.
   ventricular p.

**performance**
> cardiac p.
> left ventricular
>   systolic p.
> ventricular p.

*perfringens*
> *Clostridium p.*

**perfusion**
> cerebral p.
> p. defect
> myocardial p.
> p. pressure
> p. scintigraphy

**periaortic abscess**
**periarteritis nodosa**
**peribronchial cuffing**
**pericardectomy**
**pericardia**
**pericardiac tumor**
**pericardial**
> p. biopsy
> p. calcification
> p. cyst
> p. disease
> p. effusion
> p. fluid
> p. fremitus
> p. friction rub
> p. friction sound
> p. knock
> p. murmur
> p. poudrage
> p. pressure
> p. reflex
> p. rub
> p. tamponade
> p. teratoma
> p. window

**pericardial effusion**
> chylous p. e.
> silent p. e.

**pericardicentesis**

**pericardiectomy**
> parietal p.
> visceral p.

**pericardii**
> hydrops p.
> paracentesis p.

**pericardiocentesis**
**pericardiorrhaphy**
**pericardioscopy**
**pericardiosternal ligament**
**pericardiostomy**
**pericardiotomy**
> subxiphoid limited p.

**pericarditic**
**pericarditis**
> acute p.
> adhesive p.
> bacterial p.
> calcific p.
> cholesterol p.
> chronic constrictive p.
> constrictive p.
> drug-associated p.
> effusive-constrictive p.
> fibrinous p.
> gram-negative p.
> histoplasmic p.
> infective p.
> internal adhesive p.
> localized p.
> meningococcal p.
> neoplastic p.
> p. obliterans
> occult p.
> purulent p.
> rheumatic p.
> p. sicca
> subacute p.
> p. of systemic lupus
>   erythematosus
> transient p.
> tuberculous p.
> uremic p.

**pericarditis** *(continued)*
    p. villosa
    viral p.
**pericarditis-myocarditis**
  **syndrome**
**pericardium,** pl. **pericardia**
    absent p.
    adherent p.
    bread-and-butter p.
    congenitally absent p.
    empyema of p.
    p. fibrosum
    p. serosum
    shaggy p.
    thickened p.
**pericardotomy**
**peri-infarction block**
**perimembranous ventricular**
  **septal defect**
**perimuscular plexus**
**perimyoendocarditis**
**perimysial plexus**
**perindopril**
**perineal artery**
**period**
    absolute refractory p.
    atrial refractory p.
    diastolic filling p.
    ejection p.
    intersystolic p.
    isoelectric p.
    isometric p.
    isometric p. of cardiac
      cycle
    isovolumic relaxation p.
    postinfarction p.
    postpartum p.
    preejection p. (PEP)
    pulse p.
    refractory p.
    refractory p. of
      electronic pacemaker
    systolic ejection p.
    ventricular refractory p.

    vulnerable p.,
      vulnerable p. of heart
    Wenckebach p.
**periodic**
    p. paralysis
    p. respiration
**periorbital edema**
**periosteum**
**peripartum**
**peripheral**
    p. angioplasty
    p. arteriosclerosis
    p. atherectomy system
    p. atherosclerotic disease
    p. circulation
    p. edema
    p. pulmonic stenosis
    p. resistance
    p. resistance unit (PRU)
    p. stigmata
    p. vascular disease
    p. vascular resistance
**peristasis**
**peristatic hyperemia**
**perisystole**
**perisystolic**
**peritoneal dialysis**
**Peritrate**
**permanent**
    p. cardiac pacing lead
    p. pacemaker placement
    p. pacing
    p. pacing lead
**peroneal**
    p. artery
    p. muscular atrophy
**peroxide**
    hydrogen p.
**Per-Q-Cath percutaneously**
  **inserted central venous**
  **catheter**
**Persantine**
**persistent**
    p. atrioventricular canal

p. ductus arteriosus
p. fetal circulation
p. ostium primum
p. truncus arteriosus
**perspective**
surgical p.
**Perthes' test**
**Pertofrane**
**pertussis toxin**
**pervenous pacemaker**
**pes cavus**
**PET**
positron emission
tomography
**petechia,** pl. **petechiae**
*Petrillium*
**PFR**
peak filling rate
**phacoma**
**Phantom**
P. guide wire
P. wire
**phantom**
p. aneurysm
p. tumor
**pharmacologic stress**
**pharmacology**
**pharmacotherapy**
**pharyngeal pouch syndrome**
**pharyngitis**
**phase**
ejection p.
p. image
plateau p.
supernormal recovery p.
vulnerable p.
**phased**
p. array sector scanner
p. array sector
transducer
p. array system
p. array technology
p. array transducer
**phased array transducer**

**phasic**
p. arrhythmia
p. sinus arrhythmia
**P-H conduction time**
**phenindione**
p. sensitivity
**phenobarbital**
**phenomena**
**phenomenon,** pl. **phenomena**
AFORMED p.
Aschner's p.
Ashley's p.
Ashman's p.
Bowditch's p.
dip p.
Ehret's p.
Gallavardin's p.
gap p.
Gärtner's vein p.
Goldblatt's p.
Hill's p.
Katz-Wachtel p.
Litten's p.
no-reflow p.
Raynaud's p.
reentry p.
R-on-T p.
Schellong-Strisower p.
staircase p.
steal p.
Treppe's p.
warm-up p.
Wenckebach's p.
Woodworth's p.
**phenothiazine**
**phenoxybenzamine**
p. hydrochloride
**phentolamine**
p. hydrochloride
p. mesylate
p. methanesulfonate
**phenylbutazone**
p. sensitivity

phenylephrine
    p. hydrochloride
phenylpropanolamine
    p. toxicity
phenytoin
pheochromocytoma
*Phialophora*
phlebarteriectasia
phlebectasia
phlebemphraxis
phlebitis
phlebodynamics
phlebogram
phlebography
phlebolithiasis
phlebomanometer
phlebostasis
phlebotomy
    bloodless p.
phlegmasia
    p. alba dolens
    p. cerulea dolens
Phoenix pacemaker
phonoangiography
phonocardiogram
phonocardiograph
    linear p.
    logarithmic p.
    spectral p.
    stethoscopic p.
phonocardiographic transducer
phonocardiography
phonocatheter
phonoscope
phonoscopy
phosphate
phosphatidylcholine (PtdCho)
phosphodiesterase inhibitor
phosphofructokinase
Phosphoinositol
phosphokinase
    creatine p. (CPK)
phospholamban
phospholipid

phosphomonoesterase
phosphorus
phosphorylase
    glycogen p.
    p. kinase
phosphorylation
    oxidative p.
photoablation
photodisruption
photon
    annihilation p.
photopeak
photostethoscope
phrenic nerve
phrenocardia
phthisis
    aneurysmal p.
physical
    p. activity
    p. examination
    p. inactivity
physiodensitometry
physiologic
    p. congestion
    p. measurement
physiological
    p. measurement
    p. monitoring
    p. overreactivity
    p. split of $S_2$
    p. stress
physiology
    constrictive p.
    Eisenmenger's p.
phytanic acid accumulation
pickwickian syndrome
Picolino monorail catheter
Pierre Robin syndrome
piesis
piezoelectric
pigeon chest
pigtail catheter
Pilling microanastomosis
  clamp

pimobendan
pincushion distortion
pindolol
pink puffers
Pins'
    P. sign
    P. syndrome
piperacillin
Piperanometozine
Pipracil
pirbuterol
piretanide
Pirmentol
pirolazamide
piroximone
pistol-shot femoral sound
piston pulse
pituitary gland
P-J interval
placement
    permanent pacemaker p.
    temporary pacemaker p.
placental barrier
plane
    orthogonal p.
plant toxicity
plaque
    atheromatous p.
    atherosclerotic p.
    carcinoid p.
    fibrous p.
    Hollenhorst p.
    unstable p.
plasma
    p. coagulation system
    p. colloid osmotic
      pressure
    p. exchange column
    fresh frozen p. (FFP)
    p. volume
plasmalemma
plasmapheresis
plasmin

plasminogen
    p. activator
    p. activator inhibitor
plasminogen-streptokinase
  complex
plasmodium embolism
plastic polymer
plateau
    p. phase
    p. pulse
    ventricular p.
platelet
    p. antibody
    p. imaging
platelet-derived growth factor
platelet factor 4
platypnea
platysma
pledget
    Dacron p.
    Meadox Teflon felt p.
    polypropylene p.
    Teflon p.
Plendil
pleomorphic premature
  ventricular complex
plethora
plethysmograph
plethysmography
    impedance p.
pleura
pleural
    p. effusion
    p. fluid
    p. poudrage
pleuritic chest pain
pleuropericardial murmur
plexectomy
plexogenic pulmonary
  arteriopathy
plexus
    perimuscular p.
    perimysial p.
pliability

**P loop**
**plop**
> tumor p.

**plot**
> bull's-eye p.

**plug**
> Ivalon p.

**Plummer's disease**
**PMI**
> point of maximum impulse

**P-mitrale**
**PMV**
> percutaneous mitral balloon valvuloplasty

**PND**
> paroxysmal nocturnal dyspnea

**pneocardiac reflex**
**pneumatic**
> p. antishock garment
> p. tourniquet
> p. trousers

**pneumatocardia**
**pneumatohemia**
**pneumocyte**
**pneumohemia**
**pneumohydropericardium**
**pneumomediastinum**
**pneumonia**
> embolic p.
> eosinophilic p.

*pneumoniae*
> *Klebsiella p.*
> *Mycoplasma p.*
> *Streptococcus p.*

**pneumonitis**
> hypersensitivity p.

**pneumopericardium**
> tension p.

**pneumoplethysmography**
**pneumothorax**
> spontaneous p.

**pocket**
> pacemaker p.

**pod**
**point**
> p. of critical stenosis
> e p.
> isoelectric p.
> J p.
> p. of maximal impulse
> p. of maximum impulse (PMI)

**Poiseuille's**
> P. law
> P. resistance formula

**poisoning**
> arsenic p.
> arsine gas p.
> fluorocarbon p.
> lead p.
> mercury p.

**polarity**
**polarization**
> electrochemical p.

**polarographic method**
**poliomyelitis**
**poloxamer 188**
**polyacrylonitrile membrane**
**polyarteritis nodosa**
**polycardia**
**polychondritis**
> relapsing p.

**polycrotic**
**polycrotism**
**polycystic**
> p. kidney
> p. kidney disease
> p. tumor

**polycythemia**
> p. hypertonica
> p. vera

**polydactyly**
**polyethylene balloon**
**Poly Flex pacemaker**
**polygraph**
> Mackenzie's p.

polymer
   plastic p.
polymorphic premature
   ventricular complex
polymorphism
   restriction fragment
      length p. (RFLP)
polymorphonuclear leukocyte
polymyalgia rheumatica
   syndrome
polymyositis
polyneuritiformis
   heredopathia atactica p.
polyneuropathy
   Roussy-Lévy p.
polyostotic fibrous dysplasia
polyp
   cardiac p.
Poly-Plus Dacron vascular
   graft
polypous endocarditis
polypropylene
   p. intracardiac patch
   p. pledget
polysaccharide storage disease
polysome
polysplenia
Polystan cardiotomy reservoir
polytetrafluoroethylene (PTFE)
polythiazide
polyurethane foam
polyuria
polyvinyl
   p. chloride (PVC)
   p. chloride balloon
Pompe's disease
ponderal index
ponopalmosis
popliteal
   p. artery
   p. pulse
popping sensation
population inversion

porcine
   p. heterograft
   p. prosthesis
   p. prosthetic valve
   p. valve
pork insulin
porphyria
   acute intermittent p.
Porstmann technique
port
   side p.
Port-A-Cath implantable
   catheter system
portacaval
   p. anastomosis
   p. shunt
portal
   p. hypertension
   p. vein
   p. vein thrombosis
portion
   infradiaphragmatic p.
position
   body p.
   electrical heart p.
   heart p.
   LAO p.
   left anterior oblique p.
   levo-transposed p.
   RAO p.
   right anterior oblique p.
   Trendelenburg p.
   tricuspid p.
positioning screw
positive
   p. chronotropism
   p. end-expiratory
      pressure (PEEP)
positron emission tomography
   (PET)
postanesthesia pulmonary
   edema
postcardiotomy syndrome

postcardioversion pulmonary
   edema
postcatheterization
postcommissurotomy syndrome
postdiastolic
postdicrotic
postdrive depression
postductal
posterior
     p. approach
     p. descending artery
       (PDA)
     p. descending coronary
       artery
     p. leaflet
     p. myocardial infarction
postextrasystolic
     p. aberrancy
     p. pause
     p. potentiation
     p. T wave
postinfarction
     p. angina
     p. period
     p. syndrome
postinfectious bradycardia
postinflammatory
postintervention
postmicturition syncope
postmortem
     p. clot
     p. thrombus
postmyocardial
     p. infarction
     p. infarction syndrome
postoperative assessment
postpartum
     p. cardiomyopathy
     p. hypertension
     p. period
postperfusion
     p. lung
     p. syndrome
postpericardiotomy syndrome

postprocedural management
postpump syndrome
postrenal azotemia
postsphygmic interval
posttussive syncope
postural hypotension
posture
     Stern's p.
Potain's sign
potassium
     canrenoate p.
     p. chloride
     p. gluconate
     p. inhibition
     p. ion
     p. wasting
potassium-glucose-insulin
potassium-sparing diuretic
potential
     action p.
     maximum negative p.
     membrane p.
     resting p.
     resting membrane p.
     transmembrane p.
potentiation
     postextrasystolic p.
Potts'
     P. anastomosis
     P. operation
     P. procedure
Pott's aneurysm
Potts-Cournand needle
Potts needle
pouch
     Parsonnet pulse
      generator p.
poudrage
     pericardial p.
     pleural p.
povidone-iodine
power
     p. failure
     p. injector

left ventricular p.
resolving p.
ventricular p.
**P-P interval**
**P-pulmonale**
**P-Q interval**
**PR-AC measurement**
**practolol**
**Pravachol**
**pravastatin sodium**
**prazosin hydrochloride**
**preautomatic pause**
**pre-beta lipoprotein**
**precapillary sphincter**
**precardiac mesoderm**
**precatheterization**
**precordial**
p. A wave
p. catch syndrome
p. honk
p. leads
p. motion
p. movement
p. pulse
**precordialgia**
**precordium**
**prediastole**
**prediastolic**
**predicrotic**
**predictive value**
**predictor**
univariate p.
**prednisone**
**preductal**
**preeclampsia**
**preejection period (PEP)**
**preexcitation syndrome**
**preexisting condition**
**pregnancy**
**pregnancy-induced hypertension**
**preinfarction syndrome**
**prekallikrein**
**preload**
p. reduction

p. reserve
ventricular p.
**Premarin**
**premature**
p. atherosclerosis
p. atrial beat
p. atrial complex
p. atrial contraction
(PAC)
p. atrioventricular
junctional complex
p. beat
p. contraction
p. excitation
p. junctional beat
p. systole
p. ventricular beat
(PVB)
p. ventricular complex
p. ventricular
contraction (PVC)
**premedication**
**premonitory syndrome**
**prenalterol hydrochloride**
**prenatal diagnosis**
**prenylamine**
**prerenal azotemia**
**presbycardia**
**preshaped catheter**
**presphygmic interval**
**pressor drug**
**pressoreceptive**
**pressoreceptor reflex**
**pressosensitive**
**pressosensitivity**
reflexogenic p.
**pressure**
ankle blood p.
aortic p.
aortic pullback p.
arterial p.
atrial p.
average mean p. (AMP)
barometric p.

**pressure** *(continued)*
    blood p. (BP)
    capillary p.
    cardiovascular p.
    central venous p. (CVP)
    closure p.
    coaxial p.
    colloid osmotic p.
    continuous positive
     airway p. (CPAP)
    p. conversion
    coronary venous p.
    p. decay
    diastolic p.
    diastolic blood p. (DBP)
    diastolic filling p. (DFP)
    differential blood p.
    dynamic p.
    end-diastolic p.
    end-diastolic left
     ventricular p.
    end-systolic p.
    end-systolic left
     ventricular p.
    p. gradient
    p. half-time
    high blood p.
    hyperbaric p.
    p. injector
    intracardiac p.
    intramyocardial p.
    intrapericardial p.
    intrathoracic p.
    intravascular p.
    jugular venous p.
    left atrial p.
    left ventricular p.
    left ventricular
     diastolic p.
    left ventricular end-
     diastolic p. (LVEDP)
    left ventricular filling p.
    left ventricular
     systolic p.

    mean arterial p. (MAP)
    mean diastolic left
     ventricular p.
    mean systolic left
     ventricular p.
    p. measurement
    negative p.
    normal intravascular p.
    oncotic p.
    osmotic p.
    p. overload
    peak systolic aortic p.
     (PSAP)
    peak systolic gradient p.
    perfusion p.
    pericardial p.
    plasma colloid
     osmotic p.
    positive end-
     expiratory p. (PEEP)
    PSG p.
    pullback p.
    pulmonary p.
    pulmonary arterial p.
     (Pa)
    pulmonary artery p.
    pulmonary artery
     occlusive wedge p.
    pulmonary artery
     wedge p. (PAWP)
    pulmonary capillary p.
    pulmonary capillary
     wedge p.
    pulmonary
     hypertension p.
    pulse p.
    p. recovery
    resting p.
    right atrial p.
    right ventricular
     diastolic p.
    right ventricular
     systolic p.
    p. sling

p. stasis
systolic p.
systolic blood p.
systolic left
  ventricular p.
p. tracing
p. transducer
transmural p.
transmyocardial
  perfusion p.
venous p.
ventricular p.
ventricular filling p.
p. wave
p. waveform
wedge p.
**pressure-flow relationship**
**pressure-natriuresis curve**
**pressure-volume**
  p.-v. analysis
  p.-v. curve
  p.-v. diagram
  p.-v. relation
**presyncopal spell**
**presyncope**
**presystole**
**presystolic**
  p. gallop
  p. murmur
  p. pressure and volume
  p. thrill
**prevalence**
**prevention**
  secondary p.
**prevertebral space**
**primary**
  p. cardiomyopathy
  p. closure
  p. hypertension
  p. pulmonary
    hypertension
  p. pulmonary
    hypertension murmur

**primum**
  p. atrial septal defect
  ostium p.
  septum p.
**principle**
  Beer-Lambert p.
  Fick p.
  Frank-Straub-Wiggers-
    Starling p.
  hemodynamic p.
**Prinivil**
**P-R interval**
**Prinzmetal's angina**
**Priscoline**
**probability analysis**
**proband**
**probe**
  coronary artery p.
  Doppler velocity p.
  Gallagher bipolar
    mapping p.
  hot-tip laser p.
  nuclear p.
  Parsonnet coronary p.
  p. patency
  Radiometer p.
  scintillation p.
  transesophageal p.
**Probeta**
**probucol**
**procainamide**
  p. hydrochloride
**procaine**
  p. hydrochloride
**Procan SR**
**Procardia**
**Procardia XL**
**Procath electrophysiology**
  **catheter**
**procedure**
  Björk method of
    Fontan p.
  Blalock-Taussig p.
  Brock's p.

*Bentall*

**procedure** *(continued)*
dental p.
Fontan's p.
Jatene's p.
latissimus dorsi p.
Mustard p.
outpatient p.
Potts' p.
Rashkind's p.
Rastelli's p.
septation p.
Vineberg's p.
Waterston-Cooley p.

**processing**
film p.
signal p.

**prodromal symptom**

**prodrome**

**product**
double p.
fibrinogen
degradation p.
fibrinogen-fibrin
degradation p.
fibrin split p.
rate pressure p.

**production**
carbon dioxide p.
energy p.

**profile**
aortic valve velocity p.
deflated p.

**Profile Plus balloon dilatation catheter**

**Pro-Flo catheter**

**profunda femoris artery**

**profundaplasty**

**progeria**

**progestin**

**prognosis**

**Programalith pacemaker**

**programmability**

**programmable pacemaker**

**programmed**
p. electrical stimulation
p. stimulation

**progressive**
p. interstitial pulmonary fibrosis
p. scanning
p. systemic sclerosis (PSS)

**proiosystole**

**proiosystolia**

**projection**
anterior oblique p.
anteroposterior p.
left anterior oblique p.
left lateral p.
right anterior oblique p.

**prolapse**
mitral p.
mitral valve p. (MVP)
tricuspid valve p.

**prolapsed mitral valve syndrome**

**prolate ellipse**

**proliferation**
myxomatous p.

**prolonged Q-T interval syndrome**

**promethazine**

**Promine**

**Promine SR**

**Pronestyl**

**propafenone**

**propafenone HCl**

**propagated thrombus**

**propagation**
impulse p.

**propantheline**

**Propel**
Hi-Torque floppy with P.

**propellant**
halogenated hydrocarbon p.

**prophylactic antibiotic**
**prophylaxis**
**propranolol**
> p. hydrochloride

**propylthiouracil (PTU)**
**prostacyclin**
**prostaglandin**
> p. E
> p. E$_2$

**prostate gland**
**prosthesis**, pl. **prostheses**
> aortic p.
> Carbomedics cardiac valve p.
> cardiac valve p.
> Duromedics p.
> Golaski-UMI vascular p.
> Lillehei-Kaster cardiac valve p.
> mitral p.
> Omniscience cardiac valve p.
> porcine p.
> Starr-Edwards p.
> Starr-Edwards heart valve p.
> St. Jude heart valve p.
> vascular graft p.

**prosthetic**
> p. aortic valve
> p. cardiac valve
> p. valve
> p. valve endocarditis
> p. valve thrombosis
> p. valve vegetation

**prosthetic valve**
> ball-in-cage p.v.
> biprosthetic p.v.
> Björk-Shiley p.v.
> Braunwald-Cutter p.v.
> Hall-Kaster p.v.
> porcine p.v.
> Starr-Edwards p.v.

> St. Jude p.v.
> tilting-disk p.v.

**protamine**
> p. sulfate

**protease**
**protection**
**protective**
> p. block
> p. zone

**protein**
> p. C
> coagulation p.
> contractile p.
> Gc p.
> p. kinase
> p. kinase A
> p. kinase C
> M p.
> recognition p.
> p. S

**protein-calorie**
> p.-c. deficiency
> p.-c. malnutrition

**proteinosis**
> alveolar p.

**proteinuria**
**proteolytic enzyme**
**prothrombinase complex**
**prothrombin time**
**protocol**
> Balke p.
> Balke-Ware p.
> Bruce p.
> Bruce treadmill p.
> Global Utilization of Streptokinase and TPA for Occluded Coronary Arteries p. (GUSTO protocol)
> grievance p.
> modified Bruce p.
> Naughton p.
> Naughton treadmill p.
> standard Bruce p.

**protodiastolic gallop**
**proton**
    p. density
    p. spectroscopy
**protoveratrine A and B**
**protozoal myocarditis**
**protriptyline**
    p. hydrochloride
**pro-urokinase**
**provocative testing**
**proximal**
    p. convoluted tubule
    p. end
    p. tubule
**P-R segment**
**PRT**
  percutaneous rotational
    thrombectomy
**PRU**
  peripheral resistance unit
**Pruitt-Inahara shunt**
**Pruitt vascular shunt**
**Prussian helmet sign**
**PSAP**
  peak systolic aortic pressure
**pseudangina**
**pseudoaneurysm**
**pseudoangina**
**pseudocirrhosis**
**pseudocoarctation**
**pseudocomplications**
**pseudodiastolic**
**pseudofusion beat**
**pseudohypotension**
*Pseudomonas*
    *P. aeruginosa*
**pseudopericarditis**
**pseudotruncus arteriosus**
**pseudoxanthoma**
    p. elasticum
    p. elasticum syndrome
**PSG**
  peak systolic gradient
  PSG pressure

**P-sinistrocardiale**
*psittaci*
    *Chlamydia p.*
**psittacosis**
**psoriasis**
**PSS**
  progressive systemic
  sclerosis
**psychocardiac reflex**
**psychogenic pain**
**psychological factor**
**psychosis**
**psychosocial factor**
**psychostimulant**
**psychotherapy**
**psychotropic agent**
**PTCA**
  percutaneous transluminal
  coronary angioplasty
**PtdCho**
  phosphatidylcholine
**PTFE**
  polytetrafluoroethylene
**PTT**
  partial thromboplastin time
**PTU**
  propylthiouracil
**puff**
    veiled p.
**puffer**
    pink p.'s
**pullback pressure**
**pulmonale**
    cor p.
    P-pulmonale
    pseudo-P-pulmonale
**pulmonary**
    p. angiography
    p. area
    p. arterial pressure (Pa)
    p. arteriolar resistance
    p. arteriovenous fistula
    p. arteriovenous
    malformation (PAVM)

PSVC
paroxysmal supraventricular contraction

p. artery (PA)
p. artery bands
p. artery catheterization
p. artery occlusive
wedge pressure
p. artery pressure
p. artery stenosis
p. artery wedge pressure
(PAWP)
p. atresia
p. blood flow
p. branch stenosis
p. capillary pressure
p. capillary wedge
pressure
p. circulation
p. disease
p. edema
p. embolectomy
p. embolism
p. failure
p. fibrosis
p. function
p. function test
p. gas exchange
p. heart
p. hemosiderosis
p. hypertension
p. hypertension pressure
p. incompetence
p. infarction
p. infarction syndrome
p. insufficiency
p. murmur
p. ossification
p. pain
p. pressure
p. pulse
p. rales
p. regurgitation
p. resistance
p. scintigraphy
p. stenosis

p. systemic blood flow
ratio
p. thromboembolism
p. valve
p. valve anomaly
p. valve area
p. valve disease
p. valve
echocardiography
p. valve gradient
p. valve restenosis
p. valve stenosis
p. valve vegetation
p. valvular regurgitation
p. valvular stenosis
p. valvuloplasty
p. vascular disease
p. vascular obstruction
p. vascular obstructive
disease
p. vascular reactivity
p. vascular resistance
p. vascular resistance
index
p. vasculature
p. vasculitis
p. vasoconstriction
p. vein
p. veno-occlusive disease
p. venous connection
p. venous connection
anomaly
p. venous drainage
p. venous return
p. venous return
anomaly
p. wedge angiography
**pulmonary embolism**
air p. e.
amniotic fluid p. e.
fat p. e.
myxomatous p. e.
**pulmonic**
p. atresia

**pulmonic** *(continued)*
    p. incompetence
    p. insufficiency
    p. murmur
    p. regurgitation
    p. stenosis
    p. valve
    p. valve stenosis
    p. valvuloplasty
**pulmonocoronary reflex**
**Pulsar NI implantable**
  **pacemaker**
**pulsate**
**pulsatile flow**
**pulsating empyema**
**pulsation**
**pulse**
    alternating p.
    anacrotic p.,
      anadicrotic p.
    anacrotic limb p.
    arterial p.
    bigeminal p.
    bisferious p.
    brachial p.
    bulbar p.
    cannonball p.
    capillary p.
    carotid p.
    catacrotic p.
    catadicrotic p.
    collapsing p.
    cordy p.
    Corrigan's p.
    coupled p.
    p. curve
    p. deficit
    dicrotic p.
    dorsalis pedis p.
    p. duration
    entoptic p.
    filiform p.
    gaseous p.
    p. generator

guttural p.
hard p.
hyperkinetic p.
hypokinetic p.
incisura p.
intermittent p.
irregularly irregular p.
jugular p.
jugular venous p.
Kussmaul's
  paradoxical p.
long p.
monocrotic p.
mousetail p.
movable p.
nail p.
p. oximeter
paradoxical p.
parvus et tardus p.
pedal p.
p. period
piston p.
plateau p.
popliteal p.
precordial p.
p. pressure
pulmonary p.
quadrigeminal p.
Quincke's p.
p. rate
p. repetition
respiratory p.
reversed paradoxical p.
Riegel's p.
soft p.
tense p.
thready p.
tibial p.
tidal wave p.
p. tracing
trigeminal p.
triphammer p.
p. trisection
undulating p.

vagus p.
venous p.
vermicular p.
water-hammer p.
p. wave
wiry p.
**pulsed**
    p. Doppler
    p. Doppler
      echocardiography
    p. laser ablation
**pulsed-wave Doppler mapping**
**pulse generator**
    Medtronic p. g.
**pulse-height analyzer**
**pulseless disease**
**pulsewidth**
    atrial p.
    ventricular p.
**pulsimeter, pulsometer**
**pulsus**
    p. alternans
    p. anadicrotus
    p. bigeminus
    p. bisferiens
    p. caprisans
    p. catacrotus
    p. catadicrotus
    p. celer
    p. celerimus
    p. cordis
    p. debilis
    p. differens
    p. duplex
    p. durus
    p. filiformis
    p. fluens
    p. formicans
    p. fortis
    p. frequens
    p. heterochronicus
    p. inaequalis
    p. incongruens
    p. infrequens

p. intercidens
p. intercurrens
p. irregularis perpetuus
p. magnus
p. mollis
p. monocrotus
p. myurus
p. paradoxus
p. parvus
p. parvus et tardus
p. quadrigeminus
p. rarus
p. respiratione
  intermittens
p. tardus
p. tremulus
p. trigeminus
p. vacuus
p. venosus
**pump**
    Abbott infusion p.
    abdominothoracic p.
    balloon p.
    p. current
    p. failure
    p. function
    IMED infusion p.
    intra-aortic balloon p.
    (IABP)
    IVAC infusion p.
    Kontron intra-aortic
     balloon p.
    p. lung
    p. oxygenator
**pumpkin seeding**
**pump-oxygenator**
**puncture**
    apical left ventricular p.
    direct cardiac p.
    left ventricular p.
    transseptal p.
    venous p.
**pupils**
    Argyll Robertson p.

**Puritan**
P. Bennett ETCO2
multigas analyzer
P. Bennett ventilator
**Purkinje**
P. cells
P. conduction
P. fibers
P. system
**purpura**
anaphylactoid p.
p. fulminans
Henoch-Schönlein p.
idiopathic
thrombocytopenic p.
thrombotic
thrombocytopenic p.
**purr**
**purulent pericarditis**
**pushability**
**PVB**
premature ventricular beat

**PVC**
polyvinyl chloride
premature ventricular
contraction
**P vector**
**P wave**
**P-wave**
P-w. amplitude
bifid P-w.
**PWP monitoring catheter**
**pyelonephritis**
**pyemic embolism**
**pyloric incompetence**
**pyopneumopericardium**
**pyrazinamide**
**pyrogen reaction**
**pyrophosphate**
p. imaging
p. scintigram
**pyruvate**
p. dehydrogenase
**pyruvic acid**

# Q

**Q fever**
**Qp/Qs**
  flow ratio
**Q-RB interval**
**Q-R interval**
**QRS**
  QRS alternans
  QRS complex
  QRS interval
  QRS loop
  QRS vector
**QRS-ST junction**
**Q-S$_2$ interval**
**Q-T interval**
**quadpolar w/Damato curve**
  **catheter**
**quadrigeminal**
  q. pulse
  q. rhythm
**quadrigeminy**
**quadruple rhythm**
**quad screen format**
**Quain's degeneration**
**quality control**
**quantification**
  shunt q.

**Quénu-Muret sign**
**Questran**
**Quetelet index**
**quick prothrombin time**
**Quinaglute**
**Quinalan**
**quinaprilat**
**quinapril HCl**
**quinapril HCl**
**Quinatime**
**Quincke's**
  Q. pulse
  Q. sign
**quinethazone**
**Quinidex**
**quinidine**
  q. gluconate
  q. sulfate
**quinine**
**Quinora**
**quotient**
  respiratory q. (RQ)
**Q wave**

**R**
> gas constant
> roentgen

**racemose aneurysm**

**RAD**
> right axis deviation

**rad**
> radiation absorbed dose

**radarkymography**

**radial artery**

**radiation**
> r. absorbed dose (rad)
> r. safety
> secondary r.
> r. therapy

**radiation equivalent in man (rem)**

**radical**
> hydroxyl r.
> oxygen r.

**radiculitis**
> cervical r.

**Radifocus catheter guide wire**

**radiocardiogram**

**radiocardiography**

**radiocontrast dye**

**radiofrequency**

**radiographic technique**

**radiography**

**radioimmunoassay**

**radioisotope**

**radioisotopic study**

**radiolabeled microsphere**

**Radiometer probe**

**radionuclide**
> r. angiocardiography
> r. angiography
> r. cineangiocardiography
> r. imaging
> r. scanning
> r. study

> r. technique
> r. ventriculography

**radiopacity**

**radiopaque calibrated catheter**

**radiopharmaceutical**

**radiotracer**

**RAE**
> right atrial enlargement

**railroad track sign**

**rales**
> pulmonary r.

**Raman spectroscopy**

**ramipril**

**ramus intermedius artery**

**Rand microballoon**

**range**
> dynamic r.
> logarithmic dynamic r.

**ranging**
> echo r.

**RAO**
> right anterior oblique
> RAO angulation
> RAO position

**rapid**
> r. atrial pacing
> r. depolarization
> r. filling wave

**rapid-acquisition computer assisted tomography**

**RAS**
> rotational atherectomy system

**Rashkind**
> R. balloon technique
> R. catheter
> R. double umbrella
> R. procedure
> R. septostomy balloon catheter
> R. septostomy needle

**Rastan operation**

**Rastelli's procedure**
**rate**
  baseline fetal heart r.
  complication r.
  count r.
  critical r.
  disintegration r.
  ejection r.
  erythrocyte
    sedimentation r. (ESR)
  fetal heart r.
  flow r.
  heart r. (HR)
  magnet r.   .
  maximum flow r.
  mean normalized
    systolic ejection r.
  mortality r.
  peak diastolic filling r.
  peak filling r. (PFR)
  r. pressure product
  pulse r.
  repetition r.
  r. responsive pacing
  slew r.
  systolic ejection r.
  target heart r. (THR)
**ratio**
  aorta-left atrium r.
  cardiothoracic r.
  contrast r.
  flow r. (Qp/Qs)
  pulmonary systemic
    blood flow r.
  renal vein renin r.
  resistance r.
  sex r.
  shunt r.
  ventilation-perfusion r.
**rationalization**
**Raudilan PB**
**Raudixin**
**Raudolfin**
*Rauwolfia* alkaloid

**ray**
  beta r.
  gamma r.
  r. sum
  x-r.
**Raynaud's**
  R. disease
  R. phenomenon
  R. syndrome
**Razi cannula introducer**
**RBBB**
  right bundle branch block
**RCA**
  right coronary artery
**reaction**
  anaphylactoid r.
  cholera vaccine r.
  Eisenmenger r.
  fibrinolytic r.
  fight-or-flight r.
  inflammatory r.
  pyrogen r.
  smallpox vaccine r.
  vagal r.
  vasovagal r.
**reactive**
  r. dilation
  r. hyperemia
**reactivity**
  pulmonary vascular r.
**reagin**
**real-time echocardiography**
**Recainam**
**recanalization**
**receptor**
  adrenergic r.
  alpha r.
  beta r.
  cholinergic r.
  chylomicron remnant r.
  muscarinic r.
**receptor-operated calcium**
  **channel**

**reciprocal**
  r. beat
  r. bigeminy
  r. rhythm
**reciprocating**
  r. rhythm
  r. tachycardia
**reclosure**
**recoarctation of aorta**
**recognition protein**
**recoil wave**
**recombinant**
  alterplase r.
  r. tissue plasminogen
    activator (rt-PA)
**record**
  graphic r.
  magnetic r.
**recorder**
  event r.
  videotape r.
**recording**
  Doppler r.
  M-mode r.
  r. system
**recovery**
  pressure r.
**rectification**
  anomalous r.
  inward-going r.
**rectocardiac reflex**
**recurrence risk**
**recurrent**
  r. mesenteric ischemia
  r. mesenteric vascular
    occlusion
  r. myocardial infarction
**red**
  r. atrophy
  r. thrombus
**redistribution**
  vascular r.

**reductase**
  3-hydroxy-3-
    methylglutaryl
    coenzyme A r.
**reduction**
  afterload r.
  gradient r.
  preload r.
**redundant cusp syndrome**
**reentry**
  atrioventricular nodal r.
  AV nodal r.
  bundle branch r.
  r. phenomenon
  Schmitt-Erlanger model
    of r.
  sinus node r.
  r. tachycardia
  r. theory
  ventricular r.
**reference**
  r. electrode
  r. value
**refill**
  transcapillary r.
**reflectance oximetry**
**reflecting level**
**reflection**
**Reflex**
  R. pacemaker
  R. SuperSoft steerable
    guide wire
**reflex**
  abdominocardiac r.
  Abrams' heart r.
  r. angina
  aortic r.
  Aschner-Dagnini r.
  Aschner's r.
  auriculopressor r.
  Bainbridge r.
  Bezold-Jarisch r.
  bregmocardiac r.
  cardiac depressor r.

**reflex** *(continued)*
    carotid sinus r.
    chemoreceptor r.
    craniocardiac r.
    depressor r.
    heart r.
    Kisch's r.
    oculocardiac r.
    Pavlov's r.
    pericardial r.
    pneocardiac r.
    pressoreceptor r.
    psychocardiac r.
    pulmonocoronary r.
    rectocardiac r.
    sinus r.
    r. vasodilation
    venorespiratory r.
**reflexogenic pressosensitivity**
**reflux**
    abdominojugular r.
    esophageal r.
    r. esophagitis
    gastroesophageal r.
    hepatojugular r.
**refractoriness**
**refractory**
    r. period
    r. period of electronic
    pacemaker
**Refsum's disease**
**regimen**
    dosage r.
    exercise r.
**region**
    AN r.
    heart-forming r. (HFR)
    N r.
    NH r.
**regional anesthesia**
**Registry**
    Balloon Valvuloplasty R.
    Mansfield
    Valvuloplasty R.

**Regitine**
**regression**
    r. equation
    multiple r.
**regurgitant**
    r. fraction
    r. murmur
    r. wave
**regurgitation**
    aortic r.
    mitral r.
    pulmonary r.
    pulmonary valvular r.
    pulmonic r.
    semilunar valve r.
    tricuspid r.
    valvular r.
**rehabilitation**
    cardiac r.
    vocational r.
    work r.
**reinfarction**
**Reiter's**
    R. disease
    R. syndrome
**reject control**
**rejection**
    r. cardiomyopathy
    r. cardiomyopathy
    transplantation
**relapsing**
    r. fever
    r. polychondritis
**relation**
    diastolic pressure-
    volume r.
    end-systolic pressure-
    volume r.
    end-systolic stress-
    dimension r.
    force-frequency r.
    force-length r.
    force-velocity r.
    force-velocity-length r.

force-velocity-volume r.
interval-strength r.
length-resting tension r.
length-tension r.
pressure-volume r.
resting length-tension r.
tension-length r.
ventilation-perfusion r.
ventricular end-systolic
   pressure-volume r.

**relationship**
film density-exposure r.
Laplace r.
pressure-flow r.
stress-shortening r.

**relative**
r. cardiac volume
r. incompetence
r. risk

**relaxant**
muscle r.

**relaxation**
diastolic r.
isovolumetric r.
isovolumic r.
r. loading
stress r.
r. technique
r. time
r. time index
ventricular r.

**Relay pacemaker**

**rem**
radiation equivalent in man

**remnant**
chylomicron r.

**remodeling**

**renal**
r. angiography
r. artery
r. artery bypass graft
r. artery disease
r. azotemia
r. blood vessel

r. cortical necrosis
r. cyst
r. dialysis
r. diet
r. disease
r. failure
r. fistula
r. function
r. hypertension
r. insufficiency
r. parenchymal disease
r. transplantation
r. tuberculosis
r. vein
r. vein renin ratio

**renal-splanchnic steal**
**Rendu-Osler-Weber disease**
**Renese**
**renin-angiotensin**
r.-a. blocker
r.-a. system
**renin-angiotensin-aldosterone
   system**
**renin inhibitor**
**Renografin**
**Renografin-76**
**renography**
**renomedullary lipid**
**renoprival hypertension**
**renovascular**
r. angiography
r. hypertension
**reparative cardiac surgery**
**repeat**
r. balloon aortic
   valvuloplasty
r. balloon mitral
   valvotomy
r. balloon pulmonary
   valvuloplasty
r. revascularization
**reperfusion**
r. catheter
emergency r.

**reperfusion** *(continued)*
    r.-induced hemorrhage
    r. injury
    late r.
**repetition**
    pulse r.
    r. rate
    r. time (TR)
**repetitive monomorphic**
  **ventricular tachycardia**
**replacement**
    aortic valve r. (AVR)
    mitral valve r.
    valve r.
**repletion**
**replication**
**repolarization**
    early rapid r.
    final rapid r.
**repression**
**rescue angioplasty**
**resection**
    endocardial r.
    myotomy-myectomy-
      septal r.
    septal r.
**reserpine**
**reserve**
    cardiac r.
    coronary arterial r.
    coronary flow r.
    coronary vascular r.
    coronary vasodilator r.
    diastolic r.
    extraction r.
    heart rate r.
    preload r.
    systolic r.
    vasodilator r.
**reservoir**
    Cardiometrics
      cardiotomy r.
    cardiotomy r.
    Cobe cardiotomy r.

    Intersept cardiotomy r.
    Jostra cardiotomy r.
    Polystan cardiotomy r.
    Sci-Med extracorporeal
      silicone rubber r.
    Shiley cardiotomy r.
    William Harvey
      cardiotomy r.
**residual**
    r. gradient
    r. jet
**resin**
    anion exchange r.
    bile acid binding r.
**resistance**
    afterload r.
    aortic valve r.
    coronary vascular r.
    hydraulic r.
    peripheral r.
    peripheral vascular r.
    pulmonary r.
    pulmonary arteriolar r.
    pulmonary vascular r.
    r. ratio
    systemic vascular r.
    total pulmonary r.
    vascular r.
    vascular peripheral r.
**resolution**
    energy r.
    spatial r.
    temporal r.
**resolving power**
**resonant frequency**
**respiration**
    artificial r.
    Cheyne-Stokes r.
    cyclic r.
    periodic r.
**respiratory**
    r. arrhythmia
    r. distress
    r. distress syndrome

r. function
r. infection
r. pulse
r. quotient (RQ)
r. syncytial virus
r. tract
**Respitrace**
**response**
acute r.
chronotropic r.
Cushing pressure r.
dynamic frequency r.
fight-or-flight r.
frequency r.
giving-up-given-up r.
Henry-Gauer r.
slow r.
thyrotropin-releasing
hormone r.
vigilance r.
**response-to-injury**
r.-t.-i. hypothesis
r.-t.-i. hypothesis of
atherogenesis
r.-t.-i. theory
**rest**
r. angina
r. pain
thyroid r.
**restenosis**
aortic r.
aortic valve r.
r. lesion
mitral r.
pulmonary valve r.
tricuspid r.
**resterilization**
**resting**
r. length-tension relation
r. membrane potential
r. potential
r. pressure
r. value

**restored cycle**
**restriction**
r. endonuclease
r. fragment length
polymorphism (RFLP)
**restrictive**
r. cardiomyopathy
r. heart disease
r. lung disease
**result**
true-negative test r.
true-positive test r.
**resuscitation**
cardiac r.
cardiopulmonary r.
(CPR)
mouth-to-mouth r.
**retardation**
growth r.
mental r.
**retention**
sodium r.
water r.
**reticularis**
livedo r.
**reticuloendothelial system**
**reticulum**
sarcoplasmic r.
**retina**
**retinal**
r. artery
r. vessel
**retinopathy**
hypertensive r.
**retractor**
Cooley r.
Finochietto r.
**retrieval**
intravascular foreign
body r.
**retroconduction**
**retrograde**
r. approach

193

**retrograde** *(continued)*
- r. beat
- r. block
- r. catheter insertion
- r. catheterization
- r. conduction
- r. embolism
- r. femoral approach
- r. P wave

**retrospective genetic counseling**

**return**
- anomalous pulmonary venous r.
- r. extrasystole
- pulmonary venous r.
- systemic venous r.
- total anomalous pulmonary venous r.
- venous r.

**returning cycle**

**revascularization**
- repeat r.

**reverberation artifact**

**reversed**
- r. coarctation
- r. paradoxical pulse
- r. reciprocal rhythm
- r. shunt

**reversible ischemic neurologic debility (RIND)**

**review**
- oversight r.
- peer r.

**Reye's syndrome**

**Reynold's number**

**RFLP**
- restriction fragment length polymorphism

**rhabdomyoma**

**rhabdomyosarcoma**

**rheocardiography**

**rheology**

**RheothRx**

**rheumatic**
- r. aortitis
- r. carditis
- r. endocarditis
- r. fever
- r. heart disease
- r. mitral insufficiency
- r. mitral valve stenosis
- r. myocarditis
- r. pericarditis
- r. valvulitis

**rheumatoid**
- r. arteritis
- r. arthritis
- r. factor
- r. myocarditis

*rhodesiense*
- *Trypanosoma r.*

**rhythm**
- accelerated idioventricular r.
- accelerated junctional r.
- agonal r.
- atrial r.
- atrioventricular junctional r.
- atrioventricular nodal r., A-V nodal r., upper nodal r.
- bigeminal r.
- cantering r.
- cardiac r.
- circadian r.
- coronary nodal r.
- coronary sinus r.
- coupled r.
- r. disturbance
- ectopic r.
- escape r.
- gallop r.
- idiojunctional r.
- idionodal r.
- idioventricular r.
- junctional r.

junctional escape r.
lower nodal r.
midnodal r.
nodal r.
paced r.
pendulum r.
quadrigeminal r.
quadruple r.
reciprocal r.
reciprocating r.
reversed reciprocal r.
sinus r.
tic-tac r.
trainwheel r.
trigeminal r.
triple r.
upper nodal r.
ventricular r.

**Rhythmin**
**Rhythmonorm**
**rib**
r. approximator
r. shears
r. spreader
**ribbon**
safety r.
**ribonucleic acid (RNA)**
**ribosome**
**rickettsial myocarditis**
**riding embolism**
**Riegel's pulse**
**rifampin**
**right**
r. anterior oblique (RAO)
r. anterior oblique equivalent
r. anterior oblique position
r. anterior oblique projection
r. aortic arch
r. atrial appendage

r. atrial enlargement (RAE)
r. atrial myxoma
r. atrial pressure
r. atrial thrombus
r. atrium
r. axis deviation (RAD)
r. bundle branch block (RBBB)
r. coronary artery (RCA)
r. coronary catheter
r. heart
r. heart catheter
r. heart catheterization
r. heart failure
r. pulmonary artery (RPA)
r. ventricle (RV)
r. ventricular assist device (RVAD)
r. ventricular diastolic collapse
r. ventricular diastolic pressure
r. ventricular dimension
r. ventricular dysplasia
r. ventricular ejection fraction (RVEF)
r. ventricular failure
r. ventricular function
r. ventricular hypertrophy (RVH)
r. ventricular hypoplasia
r. ventricular infarction
r. ventricular myxoma
r. ventricular obstruction
r. ventricular outflow obstruction
r. ventricular outflow tract (RVOT)
r. ventricular systolic pressure
**right-sided heart failure**

**right-to-left shunt**
**rigor**
    calcium r.
    myocardial r. mortis
**Riley-Day syndrome**
**Riley needle**
**RIND**
    reversible ischemic
    neurologic debility
**ring**
    Carpentier r.'s
    Crawford suture r.
    Duran annuloplasty r.
    St. Jude annuloplasty r.
    vascular r.
**Ringer's lactate**
**rise time**
**risk**
    r. factor
    r. index
    recurrence r.
    relative r.
    surgical r.
**Ritchie catheter**
**ritodrine**
**Rivero-Carvallo effect**
**RNA**
    ribonucleic acid
**Ro-13-6438**
**roadmapping**
    coronary r.
**Robinson index**
**Rochester-Kocher clamp**
**Rochester-Péan clamp**
**Rocky Mountain spotted fever**
**Rodrigo equation**
**Rodriguez-Alvarez catheter**
**Rodriguez catheter**
**roentgen (R)**
**roentgenogram**
    chest r.
**roentgenography**
    chest r.

**Roger's**
    R. disease
    R. murmur
**Rogers' sphygmomanometer**
**Rolleston's rule**
**Romaña's sign**
**Romano-Ward syndrome**
**Romhilt-Estes point scoring system**
**R-on-T phenomenon**
**R-on-T premature ventricular complex**
**root**
    aortic r.
**Ross needle**
**Rotablator catheter**
**rotary atherectomy device**
**rotation**
    shoulder r.
**rotational**
    r. ablation laser
    r. angioplasty catheter
    r. atherectomy system (RAS)
    r. dynamic angioplasty catheter
**Rotch's sign**
**Roth's spot**
**Roubin-Gianturco flexible coil stent**
**Rougnon-Heberden disease**
**roundworm**
**Roussy-Lévy**
    R.-L. disease
    R.-L. polyneuropathy
    R.-L. syndrome
**route of insertion**
**routine**
    r. angioplasty
    r. right heart catheterization
**RPA**, pl. **phenomena**
    right pulmonary artery

**RQ**
   respiratory quotient
**R-R interval**
**RST segment**
**rt-PA**
   recombinant tissue
      plasminogen activator
**rub**
      friction r.
      pericardial r., pericardial
         friction r.
**rubella syndrome**
**rubeola**
**rubidium-81**
**rubidium-82**
**Rubinstein-Taybi syndrome**
**rule**
      r. of bigeminy
      Liebermeister's r.
      Rolleston's r.
      Simpson's r.
**rumble**
      diastolic r.
**Rumel**
      R. clamp
      R. thoracic forceps
**Rumel tourniquet**
**R unit**
**rupture**
      aortic r.
      balloon r.

      cardiac r.
      chamber r.
      chordae tendineae r.
      esophageal r.
      interventricular septal r.
      myocardial r.
      nonpenetrating r.
      penetrating r.
      traumatic r.
      valve r.
      ventricular septal r.
**ruptured aortic aneurysm**
**RV**
   right ventricle
**RVAD**
   right ventricular assist
      device
**RVEF**
   right ventricular ejection
      fraction
**RVH**
   right ventricular
      hypertrophy
**RVOT**
   right ventricular outflow
      tract
**R wave**
**R-wave amplitude**
**Rythmodan**
**Rythmol**

**S₁**
first heart sound
**S₂**
second heart sound
**S₃**
third heart sound
S₃ gallop
**S₄**
fourth heart sound
S₄ gallop
**sabot**
coeur en s.
s. heart
**sac**
aortic s.
lateral s.
truncoaortic s.
*Saccharomyces*
**saccular**
s. aneurysm
s. aortic aneurysm
**SACT**
sinoatrial conduction time
**saddle**
s. embolism
s. embolus
**Safe-T-Coat heparin-coated thermodilution catheter**
**safety**
s. guide wire
radiation s.
s. ribbon
**sagittal view**
**sail sound**
**salbutamol**
**salicylate**
**saline**
heparinized s.
*Salmonella*
**salt**
s. depletion syndrome
dietary s.

ethylenediaminetetraacetic
acid disodium s.
s. wasting
**salt-and-water dependent hypertension**
**Saluron**
**Salutensin**
**Salutensin-Demi**
**sampling**
blood s.
chorionic villus s.
**Sandhoff's disease**
**Sansert**
**Sansom's sign**
**saphenous**
s. vein
s. vein bypass graft angiography
s. vein cannula
s. vein graft
s. vein varicosity
**sapphire lens**
**saralasin**
**sarcoid granuloma**
**sarcoidosis**
**sarcolemma lipid**
**sarcoma**
cardiac s.
Kaposi's s.
metastatic s.
**sarcomatous tumor**
**sarcomere**
**sarcoplasmic reticulum**
**sarcosporidiosis**
**sarcotubular system**
**Sarnoff aortic clamp**
**Sarns electric saw**
**SART**
sinoatrial recovery time
**Satinsky clamp**
**saturation**
oxygen s.

**saw**
> air s.
> Sarns electric s.
> sternum s.

**SAX**
> short axis

**SBE**
> subacute bacterial
> endocarditis

**SBF**
> systemic blood flow

**scale**
> activity s.
> Borg s.
> gray s.

**scalenus**
> s. anterior syndrome
> s. anticus syndrome

**scalpel**

**scan**
> s. converter
> lung s.
> MUGA s.
> scintillation s.
> sector s.
> ventilation-perfusion s.

**Scanlan vessel dilator**

**scanner**
> computed tomography s.
> phased array sector s.

**scanning**
> duplex s.
> electronic s.
> s. format
> gated blood pool s.
> interlaced s.
> lung s.
> progressive s.
> radionuclide s.

**scarlet fever**

**scarring**

**scatter**
> Compton s.

**scattered echo**

**scattergram**

**scavenger cell pathway**

**Schapiro's sign**

**Schatz-Palmaz**
> S.-P. intravascular stent
> S.-P. tubular mesh stent

**Scheie's syndrome**

**Schellong-Strisower phenomenon**

**Schellong test**

**schistosomiasis**

**Schlichter test**

**Schmitt-Erlanger model of reentry**

**Schneider catheter**

**Schoonmaker catheter**

**Schoonmaker-King single catheter technique**

**Schott treatment**

**Schumacher aorta clamp**

**Sci-Med**
> S.-M. angioplasty catheter
> S.-M. extracorporeal silicone rubber reservoir

**scimitar syndrome**

**scintigram**
> pyrophosphate s.

**scintigraphy**
> antimyosin infarct-avid s.
> exercise s.
> infarct avid myocardial s.
> myocardial perfusion s.
> perfusion s.
> pulmonary s.
> stress thallium s.
> thallium s.
> ventilation s.

**scintillation**
> s. camera

s. probe
s. scan

**scintiscan**
technetium-99m stannous pyrophosphate s.

**scissors**
Beall s.
De Martel s.
Litwak mitral valve s.
Metzenbaum s.

**sclera**
blue s.

**scleredema**
s. adultorum
s. of Buschke

**scleroderma**

**sclerosis**, pl. **scleroses**
aortic s.
arterial s.
arteriocapillary s.
arteriolar s.
endocardial s.
multiple s.
nodular s.
progressive systemic s. (PSS)
tuberous s.
vascular s.

**sclerotherapy**

**score**   *MELD*
echo s.   *CHADS2*
jeopardy s.
wall motion s.

**scorpion**
s. sting
s. venom

**scorpionfish sting**

**screw**
positioning s.

**scrub typhus**

**scurvy**

**seagull murmur**

**second**
s. degree A-V block

s. degree heart block
s. heart sound $(S_2)$
s. messengers
s. obtuse marginal artery (OM-2)
s. through fifth shock count

**secondary**
s. cardiomyopathy
s. dextrocardia
s. prevention
s. radiation
s. thrombus

**Second International Study of Infarct Survival (ISIS-2)**

**secretor**
gene s.

**sector scan**

**Sectral**

**secundum**
ostium s.
septum s.

**sedation**

**sedative**

**seeding**
pumpkin s.

**seesaw murmur**

**segment**
P-R s.
RST s.
ST s.
Ta s.
T-P-Q s.

**segmental pressure index**

**seizure**

**Seldinger**
S. needle
S. technique

**Selecor**

**Selectan**

**selective**
s. angiography
s. arteriography

**selenium**
 s. deficiency
 s. sulfide
**self-expanding stent**
**self-guiding catheter**
**self-positioning balloon**
 **catheter**
**semidirect leads**
**semihorizontal heart**
**semilunar**
 s. valve
 s. valve regurgitation
**semivertical heart**
**senile amyloidosis**
**senility**
**Senning**
 S. intra-atrial baffle
 S. operation
**sensation**
 popping s.
**sensitivity**
 s. analysis
 atrial s.
 aureomycin s.
 chlortetracycline s.
 digitalis s.
 pacemaker s.
 paracetamol s.
 phenindione s.
 phenylbutazone s.
 sulfonamide s.
 ventricular s.
**Sensolog III pacemaker**
**sensory nerve**
 cardiac s. n.
**separation**
 aortic cusp s.
 E point-septal s. (EPSS)
**sepsis**
**septa**
**septal**
 s. artery
 s. defect
 s. hypertrophy

s. perforating arteries
s. perforation
s. resection
**septal hypertrophy**
 asymmetric s. h.
**septation**
 s. of heart
 s. procedure
**septectomy**
 atrial s.
 Blalock-Hanlon atrial s.
**septic**
 s. embolization
 s. endocarditis
 s. shock
**septomarginalis**
 trabecula s.
**septostomy**
 atrial s.
 balloon atrial s.
 blade s.
 blade atrial s.
**septotomy**
 balloon atrial s.
**septum, pl. septa**
 atrial s.
 conal s.
 interatrial s.
 interventricular s.
 intraventricular s.
 membranous s.
 s. primum
 s. secundum
 sigmoid s.
 s. spurium
 Swiss cheese
  interventricular s.
 ventricular s.
**sequela, pl. sequelae**
**sequence**
 spin-echo imaging s.
**sequestrant**
 bile acid s.

**serial**
  s. cut films
  s. dilation
**serialographic filming**
**series elastic element**
**sero-effusive**
**serological test**
**seronegative**
  **spondyloarthropathy**
**serosanguineous**
**serosum**
  pericardium s.
**serotonin**
**serotype**
  M-protein s.
**Serpalan**
**Serpasil**
*Serratia*
**serum**
  s. enzyme study
  s. glutamic-oxaloacetic
    transaminase (SGOT)
  s. sickness
**set**
  ACS percutaneous
    introducer s.
  Borst side-arm
    introducer s.
  Peel-Away introducer s.
**sex**
  s. ratio
  s. steroid
**sexual activity**
**SGOT**
  serum glutamic-oxaloacetic
    transaminase
**shadow**
  acoustic s.
**shaggy pericardium**
**shallow water blackout**
**shear**
  s. stress
  s. thinning

**shears**
  rib s.
**sheath**
  Arrow s.
  arterial s.
  carotid s.
  cordis s.
  Desilets-Hoffman s.
  s. and dilator system
  French s.
  Hemaquet s.
  introducer s.
  IVT percutaneous
    catheter introducer s.
  Mullins s.
  Mullins transseptal
    catheterization s.
  percutaneous brachial s.
  Terumo Radiofocus s.
  vascular s.
  venous s.
**sheath/dilator**
  Mullins s.
**sheathing**
  halo s.
**Sheehan and Dodge technique**
**Shekelton's aneurysm**
**shield chest**
**shift**
  axis s.
  Doppler s.
**shifting pacemaker**
*Shigella*
**Shiley**
  S. cardiotomy reservoir
  S. Tetraflex vascular
    graft
**Shiley catheter**
**shock**
  cardiogenic s.
  chronic s.
  compensated s.
  counter-s.
  declamping s.

**shock** *(continued)*
    decompensated s.
    diastolic s.
    distributive s.
    hypovolemic s.
    s. index
    irreversible s.
    s. lung
    obstructive s.
    oligemic s.
    septic s.
    systolic s.
    s. therapy
    toxic s.
    s. wave lithotripsy
**Shone's anomaly**
**short axis (SAX)**
**short-axis view**
**shortening**
    circumferential s.
    circumferential fiber s.
    fiber s.
    s. fraction
    fractional s.
    fractional myocardial s.
    myocardial fiber s.
    velocity of s.
    s. velocity
    velocity of
      circumferential fiber s.
      (VCF)
    ventricular wall s.
**Shoshin disease**
**shoulder**
    s. flexion
    s. horizontal flexion
    s. rotation
**shoulder-hand syndrome**
**shudder**
    carotid s.
**shunt**
    aorta-femoral artery s.
    arteriovenous s.
    atriopulmonary s.

    bidirectional s.
    Blalock-Taussig s.
    carotid artery s.
    s. detection
    extracardiac s.
    Glenn s.
    Gott s.
    intracardiac s.
    left-to-right s.
    Model 40-400 Pruitt-
      Inahara s.
    s. pathway
    portacaval s.
    Pruitt-Inahara s.
    Pruitt vascular s.
    s. quantification
    s. ratio
    reversed s.
    right-to-left s.
    Sundt carotid
      endarterectomy s.
    systemic to
      pulmonary s.
    Vitagraft
      arteriovenous s.
    Waterston s.
**Shy-Drager syndrome**
**sickle**
    s. cell anemia
    s. cell disease
    s. cell trait
**sickness**
    African sleeping s.
    decompression s.
    mountain s.
    serum s.
    sleeping s.
**sick sinus syndrome (SSS)**
**side**
    s. lobe
    s. lobe artifact
    s. port
    s. stretching
**siderosis**

**Sidewinder percutaneous intra-aortic balloon catheter**
**Siemens**
    S. Siecure implantable cardioverter-defibrillator
    S. ventilator
**Siemens-Elema pacemaker**
**sigmoid septum**
**sign**
    Auenbrugger's s.
    auscultatory s.
    Bamberger's s.
    Branham's s.
    Broadbent's s.
    Brockenbrough-Braunwald s.
    Brockenbrough's s.
    calcium s.
    Carabello's s.
    Carvallo's s.
    clenched fist s.
    Cruveilhier-Baumgarten s.
    Delbet's s.
    de Musset's s.
    Dorendorf's s.
    doughnut s.
    Drummond's s.
    Duroziez' s.
    E s.
    Ebstein's s.
    Ewart's s.
    Ewing's s.
    Friedreich's s.
    Glasgow's s.
    Gowers' s.
    Grocco's s.
    Hamman's s.
    Heim-Kreysig s.
    Hill's s.
    Homans' s.
    knuckle s.
    Kreysig's s.
    Kussmaul's s.
    Lancisi's s.
    Landolfi's s.
    Levine's s.
    Löwenberg's cuff s.
    Müller's s.
    Musset's s.
    Nicoladoni-Branham's s.
    Osler's s.
    Perez' s.
    Pins' s.
    Potain's s.
    Prussian helmet s.
    Quénu-Muret s.
    Quincke's s.
    railroad track s.
    Romaña's s.
    Rotch's s.
    Sansom's s.
    Schapiro's s.
    square root s.
    T s.
    Traube's s.
    Westermark s.
**signal**
    s. averaging
    Doppler s.
    magnetic resonance s.
    s. processing
**signaling**
    transmembrane s.
**Sigvaris medical stockings**
**silent**
    s. electrode
    s. gap
    s. ischemia
    s. myocardial infarction
    s. myocardial ischemia
    s. pericardial effusion
**silhouette**
    cardiac s.
**silicone**
**silk guide wire**
**silver (Ag)**

**Simon Nitinol inferior vena cava filter**
**Simpson**
    S. atherectomy catheter
    S. AtheroCath
    S. coronary AtheroCath catheter
**Simpson-Robert vascular dilation system**
**Simpson's rule**
**simvastatin**
**Sinequan**
**single**
    s. atrium
    s. balloon valvotomy
    s. balloon valvuloplasty
    s. papillary muscle syndrome
    s. ventricle
    s. ventricle malposition
**single-gene disorder**
**single-photon**
    s.-p. detection
    s.-p. emission
    s.-p. emission computed tomography (SPECT)
**single-plane aortography**
**single-vessel**
    s.-v. coronary stenosis
    s.-v. disease
**sinistrocardia**
**sinistrum**
    cor s.
**sinoatrial**
    s. block
    s. conduction time (SACT)
    s. exit block
    s. node (SN)
    s. node artery
    s. recovery time (SART)
**sinoauricular block**
**sinuatrialis**
    nodus s.

**sinus**
    aortic s.
    s. arrest
    s. arrhythmia
    s. block
    s. bradycardia
    carotid s.
    coronary s.
    s. nodal reentrant tachycardia
    s. node (SN)
    s. node artery
    s. node/AV conduction abnormality
    s. node disease
    s. node dysfunction
    s. node function
    s. node recovery time
    s. node reentry
    oblique s.
    s. pause
    s. reflex
    s. rhythm
    s. standstill
    s. tachycardia
    s. of Valsalva
    s. of Valsalva aneurysm
    s. of Valsalva aortography
    Valsalva's s.
    s. venosus
    s. venosus defect
**site**
    arterial entry s.
    entry s.
**sitting-up view**
**situational syncope**
**situs**
    s. ambiguus
    s. inversus
    s. solitus

**Size**
proximal (SMA)
spinal muscular atrophy

Multicenter Investigation
for the Limitation of
Infarct S. (MILIS)
**size**
French s.
**sizer**
Björk-Shiley heart
valve s.
Meadox graft s.
**sizing balloon**
**SK**
streptokinase
**skeletal muscle**
**skeleton**
fibrous s.
**skewer technique**
**skin heart**
**Skinny balloon catheter**
**skip graft**
**SK-Pramine**
**Skylark surface electrode**
**SLE**
systemic lupus
erythematosus
**sleep**
s. apnea
s. apnea syndrome
**sleeping sickness**
**sleeve**
**slew rate**
**Slidewire extension guide**
**sliding**
s. filament theory
s. scale method
**sling**
pressure s.
**Slinky**
S. balloon
S. balloon catheter
S. PTCA catheter
**slit ventricle syndrome**

**slope**
D to E s.
E to F s.
**slow**
s. channel
s. channel blocker
s. response
**sludging**
**smallpox vaccine reaction**
**Smart position-sensing**
catheter
**Smeloff heart valve**
**Smith-Lemli-Opitz syndrome**
**smoothing**
digital s.
**smooth-muscle cell**
**SN**
sinus node
sinoatrial node
**snake venom**
**snap**
closing s.
mitral opening s. (MOS)
opening s.
tricuspid opening s.
**snare**
s. device
s. technique
**sneeze syncope**
**snowplow effect**
$^{82}$**So**
strontium-82
**Society**
Canadian
Cardiovascular S.
**sodium**
s. bicarbonate
s. channel
cromolyn s.
dantrolene s.
dietary s.
s. ion
ioxaglate s.
s. meglumine diatrizoate

**sodium** *(continued)*
    s. meglumine ioxaglate
    mercaptomerin s.
    s. nitrite
    s. nitroprusside
    s. polystyrene sulfonate
    s. polystyrene sulfonate
      enema
    pravastatin s.
    s. retention
    thiamylal s.
    thiopental s.
    warfarin s.
**sodium-potassium exchange**
**Sofarin**
**softness**
**soft pulse**
**soldered bond**
**soldier's**
    s. heart
    s. patches
**solid angle concept**
**solitus**
    situs s.
**solubility**
    lipid s.
**Solu-Cortef**
**Solu-Medrol**
**Solus pacemaker**
**somatomedin**
**somatostatin**
**Sones**
    S. catheter
    S. coronary catheter
    S. hemostatic bag
    S. technique
**sonogram**
**Sorbitrate**
**Sorenson thermodilution**
    catheter
**soroche**
**sotalol hydrochloride**

**souffle**
    cardiac s.
    mammary s.
**sound**
    atrial s.
    cannon s.
    cardiac s.
    double-shock s.
    eddy s.'s
    ejection s.
    first heart s. $(S_1)$
    fourth heart s. $(S_4)$
    friction s.
    gallop s.
    heart s.
    Korotkoff's s.
    pericardial friction s.
    pistol-shot femoral s.
    sail s.
    second heart s. $(S_2)$
    tambour s.
    third heart s. $(S_3)$
    tic-tac s.'s
    s. wave cycle
**space**
    interstitial s.
    prevertebral s.
**SpaceLabs pulse oximeter**
**spannungs-P**
**spark erosion**
**spasm**
    arterial s.
    catheter-induced s.
    catheter-related
      peripheral vessel s.
    catheter-tip s.
    coronary s.
    coronary artery s.
    esophageal s.
    vascular s.
    venous s.
**spatial**
    s. intensity
    s. resolution

s. tracking
s. vector
s. vectorcardiography
**specificity**
**speckling**
**SPECT**
single-photon emission
computed tomography
**Spectra-Cath**
**spectral phonocardiograph**
**Spectraprobe**
**spectrophotometric oximetry**
**spectroscopy**
fluorescence s.
magnetic resonance s.
proton s.
Raman s.
**spectroscopy-directed laser**
**specular echo**
**spell**
hypercyanotic s.
hypoxic s.
presyncopal s.
tetrad s.
**Spens' syndrome**
**sphincter**
precapillary s.
**sphingolipidosis**
**sphygmic interval**
**sphygmocardiograph**
**sphygmocardioscope**
**sphygmochronograph**
**sphygmogram**
**sphygmograph**
**sphygmographic**
**sphygmography**
**sphygmoid**
**sphygmomanometer**
Mosso's s.
Rogers' s.
**sphygmomanometry**
**sphygmometer**
**sphygmometroscope**
**sphygmo-oscillometer**

**sphygmopalpation**
**sphygmophone**
**sphygmoscope**
Bishop's s.
**sphygmoscopy**
**sphygmosystole**
**sphygmotonograph**
**sphygmotonometer**
**sphygmoviscosimetry**
**spider**
s. sting
s. venom
**spike-and-dome configuration**
**spin**
s. density
s. echo imaging
**spinal**
s. anesthesia
s. muscular atrophy
**spindle**
aortic s.
His s.
**spin-echo imaging sequence**
**spin-lattice time**
**spinocerebellar**
s. ataxia
s. degeneration
**spin-spin time**
**spirochetal**
s. disease
s. infection
s. myocarditis
**spirometer**
Tissot s.
**spirometry**
**spironolactone**
**splanchnicotomy**
**splanchnic vessel**
**splenic**
s. anemia
s. flexure syndrome
**splenomegaly**
**splice**
breakaway s.

**splinter hemorrhage**
**split**
>paradoxical s. of $S_2$
>physiological s. of $S_2$

**spondylitis**
>ankylosing s. (AS)

**spondyloarthropathy**
>seronegative s.

**spontaneous pneumothorax**
**spot**
>Brushfield's s.
>café-au-lait s.
>cotton-wool s.
>hot s.
>milk s.
>Roth's s.
>tendinous s.
>ventricular milk s.
>white s.

**spot-film fluorography**
**spreader**
>rib s.

**spring**
>disk s.

**spring-loaded stent**
**spurium**
>septum s.

**sputum,** pl. **sputa**
**square root sign**
**squatting**
**SSS**
>sick sinus syndrome

**ST**
>ST junction
>ST segment
>ST segment alternans
>ST segment elevation

**stab**
>s. incision
>s. wound

**stability**
**stable angina**

**stagnant**
>s. anoxia
>s. hypoxia

**stagnation**
**staining**
>endocardial s.

**stainless**
>s. steel guide wire
>s. steel wire

**staircase phenomenon**
**standard**
>s. Bruce protocol
>s. lead
>s. needle

**standby pulse generator**
**standing**
**standstill**
>atrial s.
>auricular s.
>cardiac s.
>sinus s.
>ventricular s.

**Stanford**
>S. biopsy method
>S. bioptome

**Stanicor pacemaker**
**Stannius ligature**
**staphylococcal infection**
***Staphylococcus***
>*S. aureus*

**starch**
>hydroxyethyl s.

**Starling**
>S. cruve
>S. equation
>S. forces
>S. law of the heart
>S. mechanism

**Starr-Edwards**
>S.-E. heart valve
>prosthesis
>S.-E. mitral valve
>S.-E. prosthesis

S.-E. prosthetic valve
S.-E. valve
**stasis**, pl. **stases**
  s. cirrhosis
  pressure s.
  s. ulcer
**state**
  hyperdynamic s.
  hyperkinetic s.
**static dilation technique**
**status**
  s. anginosus
  cardiac s.
  mental s.
  neurologic s.
  work s.
**steal**
  coronary s.
  endoperoxide s.
  iliac s.
  s. mechanism
  s. phenomenon
  renal-splanchnic s.
  subclavian s.
**steal mechanism**
  coronary s. m.
**steatosis**
  s. cordis
**Steell's murmur**
**Steidele's complex**
**Steinert's disease**
**stellate ganglion**
**stenocardia**
**stenosal murmur**
**stenosis**, pl. **stenoses**
  aortic s. (AS)
  branch pulmonary
   artery s.
  buttonhole s.
  calcific nodular aortic s.
  carotid s.
  chronic aortic s.
  congenital aortic s.
  coronary s.

coronary artery s.
coronary ostial s.
discrete subaortic s.
discrete subvalvular
 aortic s.
Dittrich's s.
double aortic s.
eccentric s.
fibrous subaortic s.
fish-mouth mitral s.
geometry of s.
idiopathic hypertrophic
 subaortic s. (IHSS)
infundibular s.
left main coronary s.
left main vessel
 coronary s.
mitral s.
muscular subaortic s.
peripheral pulmonic s.
point of critical s.
pulmonary s.
pulmonary artery s.
pulmonary branch s.
pulmonary valve s.
pulmonary valvular s.
pulmonic s.
pulmonic valve s.
rheumatic mitral
 valve s.
single-vessel coronary s.
subaortic s.
subpulmonary s.
subvalvular aortic s.
supravalvular aortic s.
tricuspid s.
valvular s.
valvular aortic s.
vascular s.
**stent**
balloon-expandable s.
Carpentier s.
Cook intracoronary s.
Gianturco-Roubin s.

*nitinol AneuRx*

**stent** *(continued)*
 intravascular s.
 Medinvent s.
 Roubin-Gianturco
  flexible coil s.
 Schatz-Palmaz
  intravascular s.
 Schatz-Palmaz tubular
  mesh s.
 self-expanding s.
 spring-loaded s.
 Strecker coronary s.
 thermal memory s.
 wall s.
**step**
 Krönig's s.'s

*Promus*

**sternocleidomastoid**
**sternotome**
**sternotomy**
**Stern's posture**
**sternum saw**
**steroid**
 anabolic s.
 sex s.
**Stertzer**
 S. brachial catheter
 S. guiding catheter
**stethoscope**
**stethoscopic phonocardiograph**
**Stevens-Johnson syndrome**
**Stewart-Hamilton technique**
**STI**
 systolic time intervals
**stiff heart syndrome**
**stiffness**
 active dynamic s.
 chamber s.
 diastolic s.
 elastic s.
 muscle s.
 myocardial s.
 volume s.
**stigma, pl. stigmata**
 peripheral stigmata

**Stilith implantable cardiac pulse generator**
**Still's**
 S. disease
 S. murmur
**stimulant**
 adrenergic s.
**stimulation**
 β-adrenergic s.
 paired electrical s.
 programmed s.
 programmed electrical s.
 vagal s.
**sting**
 insect s.
 scorpion s.
 scorpionfish s.
 spider s.
 wasp s.
**St. Jude**
 St. J. annuloplasty ring
 St. J. heart valve
  prosthesis
 St. J. Medical bileaflet
  valve
 St. J. mitral valve
 St. J. prosthetic aortic
  valve
 St. J. prosthetic valve
 St. J. valve
**Stockert cardiac pacing electrode**
**stockings**
 antiembolism s.
 A-T antiembolism s.
 Bellavar medical
  support s.
 Carolon life support
  antiembolism s.
 Comtesse medical
  support s.
 Florex medical
  compression s.
 Sigvaris medical s.

TED antiembolism s.
Venofit medical
  compression s.
Venoflex medical
  compression s.
Zimmer antiembolism s.
**Stokes**
  collar of S.
**Stokes-Adams**
  S.-A. disease
  S.-A. syndrome
*Stomatococcus*
**stone heart**
**stopcock**
  three-way s.
**storm**
  thyroid s.
**straddling**
  s. atrioventricular valve
  s. embolism
**straight-back syndrome**
**straight hemostat**
**strain gauge**
**stratified thrombus**
**Strauss method**
**streak**
  fatty s.
**Strecker coronary stent**
**strenuous exercise**
**Streptase**
*Streptobacillus moniliformis*
**streptococcal**
  s. antibody
  s. infection
*Streptococcus*
  *S. pneumoniae*
**streptokinase (SK)**
  s. antibody
**streptokinase-plasminogen**
  **complex**
**streptomycin**
**stress**
  emotional s.

left ventricular s.
left ventricular end-
  systolic s.
left ventricular wall s.
mental s.
meridional wall s.
pharmacologic s.
physiological s.
s. relaxation
shear s.
tensile s.
s. test
s. testing
s. thallium-201
  myocardial perfusion
  imaging
s. thallium scintigraphy
s. thallium study
ventricular wall s.
wall s.
**stress-shortening relationship**
**stretched diameter**
**stretching**
  side s.
**stria**, pl. **striae**
**striation**
  tabby cat s.
**stripe**
  subepicardial fat s.
**stroke**
  embolic s.
  heart s.
  heat s.
  s. index
  s. output
  s. volume
  s. work
  s. work index
**strontium-82** ($^{82}$So)
**Strouhal's number**
**structure**
  wall s.
**STT changes**

**Study**
    Coronary Artery
      Surgery S. (CASS)
    European Coronary
      Surgery S.
    Framingham Heart S.
    Second International S.
      of Infarct Survival
      (ISIS-2)
    Veterans Administration
      Cooperative S.

**study**
    atrial pacing s.
    Doppler s.
    electrophysiologic s.
      (EPS)
    exercise s.
    hemodynamic-
      angiographic s.
    imaging s.
    interventional s.
    intracardiac
      electrophysiologic s.
    myocardial perfusion s.
    nuclear s.
    radioisotopic s.
    radionuclide s.
    serum enzyme s.
    stress thallium s.
    wall motion s.

**stunned myocardium**
**stunning**
    myocardial s.
**St. Vitus dance**
**stylet**
    Bing s.
    cardiovascular s.
    transmyocardial
      pacing s.
    transthoracic pacing s.
**subacute**
    s. bacterial endocarditis
      (SBE)
    s. myocardial infarction

    s. pericarditis
    s. tamponade
**subaortic stenosis**
**subclavian**
    s. arteriovenous fistula
    s. artery
    s. artery bypass graft
    s. lymphatic
    s. steal
    s. steal syndrome
    s. vein
**subcostal view**
**subcutaneous nodule**
**subendocardial**
    s. ischemia
    s. layer
    s. myocardial infarction
    s. zone
**subendocardium**
**subepicardial fat stripe**
**Sublimaze**
**submassive pulmonary**
  **embolism**
**subpulmonary**
    s. obstruction
    s. stenosis
**Subramanian clamp**
**subsarcolemma cisternae**
**subsidiary atrial pacemaker**
**substance**
    neurotransmitter s.
    paramagnetic s.
**substitutional cardiac surgery**
**substrate**
    tachyarrhythmic s.
**subtraction**
    digital s.
    functional s.
    mask-mode s.
**subvalvular**
    s. aortic stenosis
    s. mitral stenosis
    s. obstruction

**subxiphoid**
   s. area
   s. limited
     pericardiotomy
**succinate**
   hydrocortisone sodium s.
   metoprolol s.
**succinylcholine**
   s. chloride
**sucker**
   Churchill s.
   intracardiac s.
**suction**
   diastolic s.
**sudden**
   s. cardiac death
   s. death
   s. infant death
     syndrome
**sufentanil citrate**
**suicide ventricle**
**sulcus,** pl. **sulci**
   atrioventricular s.
   bulboventricular s.
   coronary s.
   interventricular s.
   s. terminalis
**sulfadiazine**
**sulfamethoxazole**
**sulfasalazine**
**sulfate**
   debrisoquine s.
   dermatan s.
   guanethidine s.
   hydroxychloroquine s.
   magnesium s.
   neomycin s.
   protamine s.
   quinidine s.
   trimethoprim s.
   vincristine s.
**sulfide**
   selenium s.
**sulfinpyrazone**

**sulfisoxazole**
**sulfonamide sensitivity**
**sulfonate**
   sodium polystyrene s.
**sulfonylurea**
**sulindac**
**sulmazole**
**sum**
   ray s.
**summation**
   s. beat
   s. gallop
   impulse s.
**Sundt carotid endarterectomy**
   **shunt**
**superdicrotic**
**superimposition**
**superior**
   s. carotid artery
   s. mesenteric artery
     syndrome
   s. mesenteric vascular
     occlusion
   s. thyroid artery
   s. vena cava (SVC)
   s. vena caval syndrome
**supernormal**
   s. conduction
   s. excitation
   s. recovery phase
**superoinferior heart**
**supertension**
**supine exercise**
**supplementation**
**supply**
   energy s.
   myocardial oxygen s.
**support**
   advanced life s. (ALS)
   cardiopulmonary s.
   Dr. Gibaud thermal
     health s.
**suppression**
   overdrive s.

**supraclavicular**
s. examination
s. fossa
**suprahisian block**
**supranormal**
s. conduction
s. excitability
**suprasternal**
s. examination
s. view
**supravalvular**
s. aortic stenosis
s. aortic stenosis-
infantile hypercalcemia
syndrome
s. aortic stenosis
syndrome
**supraventricular**
s. arrhythmia
s. ectopy
s. extrasystole
s. premature contraction
s. tachyarrhythmia
s. tachycardia (SVT)
**supraventricularis**
crista s.
**surdocardiac syndrome**
**surgery**
ablative cardiac s.
bypass s.
cardiac s.
coronary artery
bypass s.
coronary artery bypass
grafting s.
coronary bypass s.
coronary bypass graft s.
definitive s.
excisional cardiac s.
noncardiac s.
open heart s.
palliative s.

reparative cardiac s.
substitutional cardiac s.
**surgical**
s. ablation
s. perspective
s. risk
**Surgicraft**
S. pacemaker electrode
S. suture
**Surgilase 150 laser**
**Surgilon suture**
**Surgitool prosthetic valve**
**Surital**
**Surmontil**
**Survey**
Jenkins Activity S.
**suspended heart**
**susurrus**
**Sutton's law**
**suture**
chromic catgut s.
Ethibond s.
figure-of-eight s.
Mersilene s.
Nurolon s.
Surgicraft s.
Surgilon s.
Ti-Cron s.
**SVC, pl. venae cavae**
superior vena cava
**SVT**
supraventricular tachycardia
**swallowing**
**Swan-Ganz**
S.-G. bipolar pacing
catheter
S.-G. catheter
**Swank high-flow arterial
blood filter**
**S wave**
**sweating**
**sweep**
**swinging heart**

**Swiss**
S. cheese defect
S. cheese interventricular
septum
**switch operation**
**Sydenham's chorea**
**Symbios pacemaker**
**symmetric**
s. asphyxia
s. vitiligo
**sympathectomy,**
**sympathetectomy**
lumbar s.
**sympathetic nervous system**
**sympathoadrenal system**
**sympatholytic**
**sympathomimetic**
s. amine
s. drug
**symphysis,** gen. **symphyses**
cardiac s.
**symptom**
Baumès s.
Duroziez' s.
Fischer's s.
gastrointestinal s.
Kussmaul's s.
prodromal s.
Trunecek's s.
**Synapse electrocardiographic**
**cream**
**synchronization**
**Synchrony**
S. II pacemaker
S. I pacemaker
S. pacemaker
**synchrony**
atrial s.
**syncopal**
s. migraine
s. migraine headache
**syncope**
Adams-Stokes s.
carotid sinus s.

cough s.
defecation s.
deglutition s.
diver's s.
hypoglycemic s.
hypoxic s.
hysterical s.
micturition s.
migraine s.
near-s.
noncardiac s.
orthostatic s.
postmicturition s.
posttussive s.
situational s.
sneeze s.
vasodepressor s.
vasovagal s.
**syndrome**
acquired
immunodeficiency s.
(AIDS)
Adams-Stokes s.
adrenogenital s.
adult respiratory
distress s. (ARDS)
Albright's s.
Alport's s.
amniotic fluid s.
aortic arch s.
aortic arteritis s.
Apert's s.
arteriohepatic
dysplasia s.
Ask-Upmark s.
Austrian's s.
Ayerza's s.
ballooning mitral
cusp s.
Barlow s.
Bauer's s.
Behçet's s.
Bernheim's s.
Beuren s.

**syndrome** *(continued)*
- billowing mitral valve s.
- Bland-White-Garland s.
- blue toe s.
- Bradbury-Eggleston s.
- bradycardia-tachycardia s.
- Budd-Chiari s.
- carcinoid s.
- cardiofacial s.
- carotid sinus s.
- cervical rib s.
- Charcot-Weiss-Baker s.
- CHARGE association s.
- Churg-Strauss s.
- click murmur s.
- Cockayne's s.
- Cogan's s.
- Conn's s.
- Conradi-Hünermann s.
- Cornelia de Lange s.
- costochondral s.
- costoclavicular rib s.
- costosternal s.
- cri du chat s.
- Cushing's s.
- cutis laxa s.
- DaCosta's s.
- de Lange's s.
- DiGeorge s.
- Down's s.
- Dressler's s.
- effort s.
- Ehlers-Danlos s.
- Eisenmenger's s.
- Ellis-van Creveld s.
- euthyroid sick s.
- fetal alcohol s. (FAS)
- floppy valve s.
- Forney's s.
- Gaisböck's s.
- gastrocardiac s.
- Gorlin's s.
- Gowers' s.
- Grönblad-Strandberg s.
- Guillain-Barré s.
- Hamman-Rich s.
- Hegglin's s.
- Henoch-Schönlein s.
- holiday heart s.
- Holt-Oram s.
- homocystinuria s.
- Hughes-Stovin s.
- Hunter's s.
- Hurler's s.
- hyperabduction s.
- hypereosinophilic s.
- hyperkinetic heart s.
- hypersensitive carotid sinus s.
- hyperviscosity s.
- hypoplastic left heart s. (HLHS)
- incontinentia pigmenti s.
- intermediate s.
- Jervell and Lange-Nielsen s.
- Kallmann's s.
- Kartagener's s.
- Kearns' s.
- Kearns-Sayre s.
- Klinefelter's s.
- Klippel-Feil s.
- Klippel-Trenaunay-Weber s.
- Kugelberg-Welander s.
- LAMB s.
- Landouzy-Déjérine s.
- Laurence-Moon-Bardet-Biedl s.
- Laurence-Moon-Biedl s.
- Lenègre's s.
- LEOPARD s.
- Leriche's s.
- Lev's s.
- Libman-Sacks s.
- Löffler's s.
- long Q-T s.

Lown-Ganong-Levine s.
low salt s., low
   sodium s.
Lutembacher's s.
malignant carcinoid s.
Mallory-Weiss s.
Marfan's s.
Maroteaux-Lamy s.
Martorell's s.
McArdle's s.
Meadows' s.
metastatic carcinoid s.
midsystolic click s.
mitral valve prolapse s.
Mondor's s.
Morgagni-Adams-
   Stokes s.
Morquio's s.
mucocutaneous lymph
   node s.
multiple lentigines s.
myocardial ischemic s.
NAME s.
nephrotic s.
Noonan's s.
obesity-hypoventilation s.
oculomucocutaneous s.
Osler-Weber-Rendu s.
Paget-von Schrötter s.
papillary muscle s.
pericarditis-myocarditis s.
pharyngeal pouch s.
pickwickian s.
Pierre Robin s.
Pins' s.
polymyalgia
   rheumatica s.
postcardiotomy s.
postcommissurotomy s.
postinfarction s.
postmyocardial
   infarction s.
postperfusion s.
postpericardiotomy s.

postpump s.
precordial catch s.
preexcitation s.
preinfarction s.
premonitory s.
prolapsed mitral
   valve s.
prolonged Q-T
   interval s.
pseudoxanthoma
   elasticum s.
pulmonary infarction s.
Raynaud's s.
redundant cusp s.
Reiter's s.
respiratory distress s.
Reye's s.
Riley-Day s.
Romano-Ward s.
Roussy-Lévy s.
rubella s.
Rubinstein-Taybi s.
salt depletion s.
scalenus anterior s.
scalenus anticus s.
Scheie's s.
scimitar s.
shoulder-hand s.
Shy-Drager s.
sick sinus s. (SSS)
single papillary
   muscle s.
sleep apnea s.
slit ventricle s.
Smith-Lemli-Opitz s.
Spens' s.
splenic flexure s.
Stevens-Johnson s.
stiff heart s.
Stokes-Adams s.
straight-back s.
subclavian steal s.
sudden infant death s.

219

**syndrome** *(continued)*
superior mesenteric
artery s.
superior vena caval s.
supravalvular aortic
stenosis s.
supravalvular aortic
stenosis-infantile
hypercalcemia s.
surdocardiac s.
systolic click-murmur s.
tachycardia-
bradycardia s.
Takayasu's s.
TAR s.
Taussig-Bing s.
thoracic outlet s.
thrombocytopenia-absent
radius s.
Tietze's s.
Treacher Collins s.
Trousseau's s.
Turner's s.
twiddler's s.
vasculocardiac s. of
hyperserotonemia
vasovagal s.
VATER association s.
velocardiofacial s.
vena caval s.
Watson's s.
Weber-Osler-Rendu s.
Werner's s.
West's s.
Williams s.
Wolff-Parkinson-White s.
s. X
XO s.
XXXX s.
XXXY s.
**synechia,** pl. **synechiae**
s. pericardii
**synthase**
glycogen s.

**synthetase**
pantothenate s.
**synvinolin**
**syphilis**
cardiovascular s.
tertiary s.
**syphilitic**
s. aneurysm
s. aortic aneurysm
s. aortic valvulitis
s. aortitis
s. myocarditis
**syringe**
Namic angiographic s.
**systaltic**
**System**
Alcon Closure S. (ACS)
**system**
adenylate cyclase s.
adrenergic nervous s.
ANCOR imaging s.
automatic exposure s.
autonomic nervous s.
Bard percutaneous
cardiopulmonary
support s.
brachiocephalic s.
cardiac conduction s.
cardiovascular s.
catheter s.
catheter-snare s.
catheter-tip
micromanometer s.
cine pulse s.
circulatory s.
circulatory support s.
complement s.
complete pacemaker
patient testing s.
(CPTS)
conduction s.
coordinate s.
dilator-sheath s.

echocardiographic
scoring s.
electrode s.
endocrine s.
Estes point s.
expert s.
fiber optic catheter
delivery s.
fibrinolytic s.
Frank lead s.
gated s.
hexaxial reference s.
His-Purkinje s.
hospital information s.
isocenter s.
kallikrein-bradykinin s.
King double umbrella
closure s.
Lastac s.
lead s.
Medi-Tech catheter s.
micromanometer
catheter s.
Mobin-Uddin filter s.
Mullins sheath s.
nervous s.
orthogonal lead s.
Paceart complete
pacemaker patient
testing s.
parasympathetic s.
parasympathetic
nervous s.
peripheral
atherectomy s.
phased array s.
plasma coagulation s.
Port-A-Cath implantable
catheter s.
Purkinje s.
recording s.
renin-angiotensin s.
renin-angiotensin-
aldosterone s.

reticuloendothelial s.
Romhilt-Estes point
scoring s.
rotational atherectomy s.
(RAS)
sarcotubular s.
sheath and dilator s.
Simpson-Robert vascular
dilation s.
sympathetic nervous s.
sympathoadrenal s.
T s.
transluminal lysing s.
triaxial reference s.
Vario s.
vessel occlusion s.
video s.
White s. for pediatric
percutaneous
catheterization
x-ray s.

**systemic**
s. blood flow (SBF)
s. circulation
s. collateral
s. heart
s. hemodynamic
parameters
s. hemodynamics
s. hypertension
s. infection
s. lupus erythematosus
(SLE)
s. to pulmonary shunt
s. vascular resistance
s. vascular resistance
index
s. venous return

**systemic-to-pulmonary**
s.-t.-p. artery
anastomosis
s.-t.-p. connection

**systole**
aborted s.

**systole** *(continued)*
  s. alternans
  atrial s.
  auricular s.
  electromechanical s.
  late s.
  premature s.
  ventricular s.
**systolic**
  s. apical impulse
  s. blood pressure
  s. click
  s. click-murmur
    syndrome
  s. current
  s. current of injury
  s. doming
  s. ejection period
  s. ejection rate
  s. function
  s. gallop
  s. gradient
  s. heart failure
  s. honk
  s. hypertension
  s. left ventricular
    pressure
  s. motion
  s. murmur
  s. pressure
  s. pressure-time index
  s. regurgitant murmur
  s. reserve
  s. shock
  s. thrill
  s. time intervals (STI)
  s. whoop
**systolometer**

# T

**T**
>tesla

**T2**
>T. relaxation time
>T. weighted image

**T₄**
>thyroxine

**T1 weighted image**

**TA**
>tantalum

**¹⁷⁸TA**
>tantalum-178

**tabby cat striation**

**tache**
>t. blanche
>t. laiteuse

**tachyarrhythmia**
>supraventricular t.
>ventricular t.

**tachyarrhythmic substrate**

**tachycardia**
>antidromic t.
>atrial t. (AT)
>atrial chaotic t.
>atrioventricular junctional reciprocating t.
>atrioventricular nodal t., A-V nodal t.
>atrioventricular nodal reentrant t.
>atrioventricular reciprocating t., AV reciprocating t.
>auricular t.
>bidirectional ventricular t.
>bundle branch reentrant t.
>chaotic t.
>circus movement t.
>Coumel's t.

>double t.
>ectopic t.
>ectopic atrial t.
>t. en salves
>entrainment of t.
>essential t.
>t. exophthalmica
>fetal t.
>incessant t.
>multifocal t.
>nodal t.
>nonparoxysmal t.
>nonparoxysmal atrioventricular junctional t.
>nonparoxysmal junctional t.
>orthodromic t.
>paroxysmal t.
>paroxysmal atrial t. (PAT)
>paroxysmal junctional t.
>paroxysmal nodal t.
>paroxysmal reentrant supraventricular t.
>paroxysmal supraventricular t.
>t. pathway mapping
>reciprocating t.
>reentry t.
>repetitive monomorphic ventricular t.
>sinus t.
>sinus nodal reentrant t.
>supraventricular t. (SVT)
>ventricular t.
>wide-complex t.
>wide QRS t.
>t. window

**tachycardia-bradycardia syndrome**

**tachycardiac**

**tachycardia-dependent
  aberrancy**
**tachycrotic**
**tachypacing**
**tachypnea**
**tachyrhythmia**
**tachysystole**
**Takayasu-Ohnishi disease**
**Takayasu's**
  T. arteritis
  T. disease
  T. syndrome
**talc operation**
**Tambocor**
**tambour sound**
**TAMI**
  thrombolysis and
    angioplasty in myocardial
    infarction
**tamponade, tamponage**
  acute t.
  atypical t.
  cardiac t.
  low-pressure t.
  pericardial t.
  subacute t.
  traumatic t.
**tandem lesion**
**Tangier disease**
**tantalum (TA)**
**tantalum-178 ($^{178}$TA)**
**tap**
  mitral t.
**tape**
  umbilical t.
**tapered movable core curved
  wire guide**
**tapeworm**
**TAR**
  thrombocytopenia-absent
    radius
    TAR syndrome
**tardive cyanosis**

**tardus**
  pulsus t.
**target heart rate (THR)**
**tartrate**
  metoprolol t.
**Ta segment**
**taurinum**
  cor t.
**Taussig-Bing**
  T.-B. anomaly
  T.-B. disease
  T.-B. heart
  T.-B. syndrome
**Tay-Sachs disease**
**TBV**
  total blood volume
**Tc**
  technetium
**$^{99m}$Tc**
  technetium-99m
    $^{99m}$Tc imaging
**T cell**
**TCG**
  time compensation gain
**TE**
  echo delay time
**tear**
  intimal t.
  medial t.
**teardrop heart**
**TEC**
  transluminal extraction-
    endarterectomy catheter
**technetium (Tc)**
**technetium-99m ($^{99m}$Tc)**
  t.-99m imaging
  t.-99m stannous
    pyrophosphate
    scintiscan
**technique**
  ablative t.
  Amplatz t.
  antegrade/retrograde
    cardioplegia t.

atrial-well t.
bootstrap two-vessel t.
catheterization t.
clearance t.
coronary flow reserve t.
Creech t.
cutdown t.
digital subtraction t.
dilator and sheath t.
direct insertion t.
Doppler t.
Dotter t.
Douglas bag t.
entangling t.
Fick t.
flush t.
forward triangle t.
grabbing t.
Grüntzig t.
human catheterization t.
human coronary
 angiography t.
indicator dilution t.
indocyanine green
 indicator dilution t.
Judkins t.
kissing balloon t.
McGoon t.
Merendino t.
modified brachial t.
multipurpose t.
percutaneous t.
Porstmann t.
radiographic t.
radionuclide t.
Rashkind balloon t.
Rashkind's balloon t.
relaxation t.
Schoonmaker-King single
 catheter t.
Seldinger t.
Sheehan and Dodge t.
skewer t.
snare t.

Sones t.
static dilation t.
Stewart-Hamilton t.
thermal dilution t.
thermodilution t.
velocity catheter t.
**technology**
 phased array t.
**TED antiembolism stockings**
**TEDD**
 total end-diastolic diameter
**TEE**
 transesophageal
 echocardiography
**Tefcor movable core straight
 wire guide**
**Teflon**
 T. coating
 T. intracardiac patch
 T. pledget
 T. pledget suture
 buttress
**Teflon-coated guide wire**
**telangiectasia**, pl. **telangiectases**
 hemorrhagic t.
 hereditary
 hemorrhagic t.
**telecardiogram**
**telecardiophone**
**telectronic leads**
**Telectronics ATP implantable
 cardioverter-defibrillator**
**telediastolic**
**telelectrocardiogram**
**telemetry**
 cardiac t.
**telesystolic**
**temperature, pulse, and
 respiration (TPR)**
**temporal**
 t. arteritis
 t. dispersion
 t. resolution

**temporary**
>  t. pacemaker placement
>  t. pacing
>  t. pervenous lead

**Tenathan**

**tendineae**
>  chorda t., pl. chordae t.

**tendinosum**
>  xanthoma t.

**tendinous**
>  t. spot
>  t. xanthoma

**tendon**
>  false t.

**tendophony**

**Tenif**

**tenonometer**

**tenophony**

**Tenormin**

**tense pulse**

**tensile stress**

**Tensilon**

**tension**
>  alveolar t.
>  carbon dioxide t.
>  left ventricular t.
>  myocardial t.
>  oxygen t.
>  t. pneumopericardium
>  wall t.

**tension-length relation**

**tension-time index**

**teratoma**
>  pericardial t.
>  t. tumor

**terazosin hydrochloride**

**terbutaline**

**terminal**
>  t. cisternae
>  t. endocarditis
>  t. groove
>  t. Purkinje fibers
>  Wilson central t.

**terminalis**
>  crista t.
>  sulcus t.

**tertiary syphilis**

**Terumo**
>  T. guide wire
>  T. "m" wire
>  T. Radiofocus sheath

**TESD**
>  total end-systolic diameter

**tesla (T)**

**test**
>  acetylcholine t.
>  acid infusion t.
>  adenosine thallium t.
>  Allen t.
>  anoxemia t.
>  ASTZ t.
>  atrial pacing stress t.
>  atropine t.
>  Balke-Ware t.
>  Bernstein t.
>  blood t.
>  breath-holding t.
>  cold pressor t.
>  complement-fixation t.
>  Crampton t.
>  Dehio's t.
>  dexamethasone
>    suppression t.
>  electrophysiologic t.
>  ergonovine t.
>  ergonovine
>    provocation t.
>  ether t.
>  exercise t.
>  exercise stress t. (EST)
>  exercise tolerance t.
>  hepatojugular reflux t.
>  hypoxemia t.
>  isoproterenol stress t.
>  Machado-Guerreiro t.
>  Master's t., Master's
>    two-step exercise t.

*D-dimer*

methacholine t.
Pachon's t.
Perthes' t.
pulmonary function t.
Schellong t.
Schlichter t.
serological t.
stress t.
thallium stress t.
thallium-201 stress t.
thyroid function t.
tilt-table t.
tolazoline t.
treadmill t.
Trendelenburg's t.
two-step exercise t.
Valsalva t.
VDRL t.
volume-challenge t.

**testimony**
expert t.

**testing**
apex impulse t.
cold pressor t.
diagnostic t.
laboratory t.
noninvasive t.
provocative t.
stress t.

**testosterone**
**tetanus**
**tetracaine hydrochloride**
**tetracrotic**
**tetracycline**
**tetrad**
Fallot's t.
t. spell

**tetralogy**
Eisenmenger's t.
t. of Fallot
Fallot's t.

**tetranitrate**
erythrityl t.
pentaerythritol t.

**tetrodotoxin**
**TGC**
time-varied gain control
**TGF**
transforming growth factor
**TGV, pl. arteries**
transposition of great vessels
**thalassemia**
**thalidomide**
**Thalitone**
**thallium (Tl)**
t. imaging
t. perfusion imaging
t. scintigraphy
t. stress test
**thallium-201 ($^{201}$Tl)**
**thallium-201 stress test**
**thebesian**
t. foramina
t. valve
t. vein
**theobromine, pl. arteries**
**theophylline**
**theorem**
Bayes' t.
Bernoulli's t.
**theory**
Bayliss t.
Cannon's t.
cross-linkage t.
dipole t.
immunological t.
myogenic t.
neuroendocrine t.
neurogenic t.
reentry t.
response-to-injury t.
sliding filament t.
**therapeutic endpoint**
**therapy**
antiarrhythmic t.
anticoagulant t.
antiplatelet t.
behavioral t.

**therapy** *(continued)*
    electroconvulsive t.
    embolization t.
    fibrinolytic t.
    immunosuppressive t.
    medical t.
    oral anticoagulant t.
    oxygen t.
    radiation t.
    shock t.
    thrombolytic t.
    warfarin t.
**thermal**
    t. dilution technique
    t. memory stent
**thermistor**
**thermodilution**
    t. balloon catheter
    t. cardiac output
    t. catheter
    t. catheter introducer kit
    coronary sinus t.
    t. kit
    t. measurement
    t. method
    t. output
    t. technique
**thermoplastic**
**thiamine deficiency**
**thiamylal sodium**
**thiazide diuretic**
**thickened pericardium**
**thickening**
    cardiac wall t.
    diffuse intimal t.
    leaflet t.
    wall t.
**thickness**
    wall t.
**thinning**
    shear t.
    ventricular wall t.
**thin-walled needle**
**thioamide**

**thiocyanate**
**Thiomerin**
**thionamide**
**thiopental**
    t. sodium
**thioridazine**
    t. hydrochloride
**third**
    t. degree heart block
    t. heart sound (S$_3$)
**Thoma's ampulla**
**Thomsen's disease**
**thoracentesis**
**thoracic**
    t. aorta
    t. aortic aneurysm
    t. duct
    t. nerve
    t. outlet syndrome
    t. vessel
**thoracis**
    paracentesis t.
**thoracoabdominal aortic aneurysm**
**thoracotomy incision**
**thorax**
**Thorazine**
**THR**
    target heart rate
**thready pulse**
**three-dimensional echocardiography**
**three-sign**
**three-way stopcock**
**threshold**
    anaerobic t.
    atrial capture t.
    fibrillation t.
    lactate t.
    ventilatory t.
    ventricular capture t.
    work t.
**thrill**
    diastolic t.

presystolic t.
systolic t.
**throb**
**thrombasthenia**
**thrombectomy**
    percutaneous
      rotational t. (PRT)
**thrombi**
**thrombin time (TT)**
**thromboangiitis**
    t. obliterans
**thromboaortopathy**
    occlusive t.
**thromboarteritis**
**thromboclasis**
**thromboclastic**
**thrombocytopenia**
**thrombocytopenia-absent radius
  (TAR)**
**thrombocytopenia-absent radius
  syndrome**
**thrombocytosis**
**thromboelastogram**
**thromboembolic disease**
**thromboembolism**
    pulmonary t.
    venous t.
**thromboendocarditis**
**thromboglobulin**
    beta t.
**thromboid**
**thrombolic**
**thrombolus**
**thrombolysis**
    t. and angioplasty in
      myocardial infarction
      (TAMI)
    coronary t.
**thrombolytic**
    t. agent
    t. therapy
**thrombomodulin**

**thrombophlebitis**
    t. migrans
    t. saltans
**thromboplastin**
    partial t. time (PTT)
    t. time
**thrombosed**
**thrombosis, pl. thromboses**
    aortic t.
    aortoiliac t.
    arterial t.
    atrophic t.
    brachial artery t.
    cerebral t.
    cerebrovascular t.
    compression t.
    coronary t.
    coronary artery t.
    creeping t.
    deep venous t. (DVT)
    dilation t.
    effort t.
    femoral artery t.
    femoral venous t.
    iliac vein t.
    jumping t.
    laser-induced t.
    marantic t., marasmic t.
    mural t.
    portal vein t.
    prosthetic valve t.
    venous t.
**thrombostasis**
**thrombotic**
    t. microangiopathy
    t. thrombocytopenic
      purpura
**thromboxane**
    t. receptor antagonist
    t. synthetase inhibitor
**thromboxane $A_2$**
**thrombus, pl. thrombi**
    agglutinative t.
    agonal t.

**thrombus** *(continued)*
  antemortem t.
  atrial t.
  ball t.
  ball-valve t.
  fibrin t.
  globular t.
  hyaline t.
  intracardiac t.
  laminated t.
  left atrial t.
  marantic t., marasmic t.
  mixed t.
  mural t.
  obstructive t.
  pale t.
  parietal t.
  postmortem t.
  propagated t.
  red t.
  right atrial t.
  secondary t.
  stratified t.
  valvular t.
  ventricular t.
  white t.
**through-and-through**
  **myocardial infarction**
**Thruflex balloon**
**thumpversion**
**thymoma**
**thyrocardiac disease**
**thyroid**
  t. antibody
  t. bruit
  t. disease
  t. function test
  t. gland
  t. hormone
  t. rest
  t. storm
  t. tumor
**thyroiditis**
**thyroid-stimulating hormone**

**thyrotoxic heart disease**
**thyrotoxicosis**
**thyrotropin**
**thyrotropin-releasing hormone**
  **response**
**thyroxine, thyroxin (T$_4$)**
D-**thyroxine**
L-**thyroxine**
**TIA**
  transient ischemic attack
**tiapamil**
**Tibbs arterial cannula**
**tibial**
  t. artery
  t. pulse
**ticarcillin**
**tick paralysis**
**Ticlid**
**ticlopidine HCl**
**Ti-Cron suture**
**tic-tac**
  t.-t. rhythm
  t.-t. sounds
**tidal**
  t. wave
  t. wave pulse
**Tietze's syndrome**
**tiger heart**
**tight junction**
**tilting-disk**
  t.-d. occluder
  t.-d. prosthetic valve
  t.-d. valve
**tilt-table test**
**time**
  acceleration t.
  activated partial
    thromboplastin t.
    (APTT, AtPP)
  A-H conduction t.
  capacitor forming t.
  charge t.
  circulation t.
  coagulation t.

t. compensation gain
  (TCG)
conduction t.
dead t.
echo delay t. (TE)
ejection t.
H-R conduction t.
H-V conduction t.
intra-atrial conduction t.
left ventricular
  ejection t. (LVET)
lysis t.
magnetic relaxation t.
P-A conduction t.
partial thromboplastin t.
  (PTT)
P-H conduction t.
prothrombin t.
quick prothrombin t.
relaxation t.
repetition t. (TR)
rise t.
sinoatrial conduction t.
  (SACT)
sinoatrial recovery t.
  (SART)
sinus node recovery t.
spin-lattice t.
spin-spin t.
thrombin t. (TT)
thromboplastin t.
T2 relaxation t.
**time-activity curve**
**time-gain-compensation**
**time-varied**
  t.-v. gain (TVG)
  t.-v. gain control (TGC)
**Timolide**
**timolol**
  t. maleate
**tip**
  Luer-Lok needle t.
  t. occluder

**tip-deflecting wire**
**Tissot spirometer**
**tissue**
  t. ablation
  adipose t.
  connective t.
  t. factor
  His-Purkinje t.
  myocardial t.
  t. necrosis
  nodal t.
  t. plasminogen activator
    (tPA, t-PA)
**tissue plasminogen activator**
  **(tPA, t-PA)**
**titer**
  antiheart antibody t.
  bactericidal t.
**Tl**
  thallium
**$^{201}$Tl**
  thallium-201
**T loop**
**TNF**
  tumor necrosis factor
**to-and-fro murmur**
**tobacco heart**
**tobramycin**
**tocainide**
**Tofranil**
**tolazoline**
  t. hydrochloride
  t. test
**tolerance**
  hemodynamic t.
**tomography**
  cine computed t.
  computed t. (CT)
  gated computed t.
  positron emission t.
    (PET)
  rapid-acquisition
    computer assisted t.

**tomography** *(continued)*
    single-photon emission computed t. (SPECT)
    ultrafast computed t.
    x-ray cine computed t.
**tone**
    Traube's double t.
**Tonocard**
**tonometer**
    Gärtner's t.
**tonometry**
**tonoscillograph**
**tonsillitis**
**tonsilloadenoidectomy**
**Toprol XL**
**Torktherm torque control catheter**
**toroidal valve**
**torque**
    t. control
    t. control balloon catheter
**Torricelli's**
    T. law
    T. orifice equation
**torsade de pointes**
*Torulopsis glabrata*
**torus aorticus**
**Toshiba biplane transesophageal transducer**
**tosylate**
    bretylium t.
**total**
    t. acidity
    t. alternans
    t. anomalous pulmonary venous connection
    t. anomalous pulmonary venous return
    t. artificial heart
    t. blood volume (TBV)
    t. circulatory arrest
    t. end-diastolic diameter (TEDD)

    t. end-systolic diameter (TESD)
    t. patient shock count
    t. pulmonary resistance
**tourniquet**
    Esmarch t.
    pneumatic t.
    Rumel t.
**toxemia**
**toxic**
    t. agent
    t. shock
**toxicity**
    amphetamine t.
    anthracycline t.
    antimony t.
    dextroamphetamine t.
    emetine t.
    fluoride t.
    hydrocarbon t.
    phenylpropanolamine t.
    plant t.
**toxin**
    t. exposure
    pertussis t.
*Toxocara canis*
**toxoplasmosis**
**tPA, t-PA**
    tissue plasminogen activator
**T-P-Q segment**
**TPR**
    temperature, pulse, and respiration
**TR**
    repetition time
**trabeculae carneae**
**trabecula septomarginalis**
**trace metal**
**tracer**
**trachea**
    bifurcation of t.
**tracheal**
    t. intubation
    t. tug

**tracheophonesis**
*trachomatis*
    *Chlamydia t.*
**tracing**
    apex impulse t. (ACG)
    carotid pulse t.
    jugular venous pulse t.
    pressure t.
    pulse t.
**trackability**
**Tracker soft stream side hole microinfusion catheter**
**tracking**
    spatial t.
**Tracrium**
**tract**
    atriohisian t.
    bypass t.
    concealed bypass t.
    gastrointestinal t.
    inflow t.
    James t.'s
    left ventricular
      outflow t. (LVOT)
    nodoventricular t.
    outflow t.
    respiratory t.
    right ventricular
      outflow t. (RVOT)
    Wolff-Parkinson-White
      bypass t.
**traction aneurysm**
**trailing edge**
**training effect**
**trainwheel rhythm**
**trait**
    sickle cell t.
**Trandate**
**trandolapril**
**tranquilizer**
**transaminase**
    glutamic-oxaloacetic t.
    (GOT)

    serum glutamic-
      oxaloacetic t. (SGOT)
**transaortic valve gradient**
**transcapillary refill**
**transcatheter**
    t. closure
    t. embolization
**transcutaneous echo**
**Transderm**
**transdermal patch**
**Transderm-Nitro**
**transducer**
    annular array t.
    t. aperture
    diaphragm t.
    Doppler t.
    echocardiographic t.
    Mikro-Tip t.
    Millar t.
    Millar Mikro-Tip
      catheter pressure t.
    Pedoff continuous
      wave t.
    phased array t.
    phased array sector t.
    phonocardiographic t.
    pressure t.
    Toshiba biplane
      transesophageal t.
**transesophageal**
    t. echo
    t. echocardiography
    (TEE)
    t. probe
**transferase**
**transform**
    Fourier t.
**transforming growth factor (TGF)**
**transfusion**
**transfusional hemosiderosis**
**transient**
    calcium t.
    t. depolarization

**transient** *(continued)*
  t. heart block
  t. inward current
  t. ischemia
  t. ischemic attack (TIA)
  t. mesenteric ischemia
  t. pericarditis
**transitional**
  t. cell
  t. cell zone
**translumbar aortography**
**transluminal**
  t. angioplasty
  t. angioplasty catheter
  t. coronary angioplasty
  t. extraction catheter
  t. extraction-
    endarterectomy catheter
    (TEC)
  t. lysing system
**transmembrane**
  t. potential
  t. signaling
  t. voltage
**transmission**
  genetic t.
**transmural**
  t. myocardial infarction
  t. pressure
**transmyocardial**
  t. pacing stylet
  t. perfusion pressure
**transplant**
  heart t.
  heart-lung t.
**transplantation**
  allogeneic t.
  bone marrow t.
  cardiac t.
  heterologous cardiac t.
  heterotopic cardiac t.
  homologous cardiac t.
  orthotopic cardiac t.

  rejection
  cardiomyopathy t.
  renal t.
**transport**
  patient t.
**transposition**
  t. of arterial stems
  t. assessment
  t. complex
  t. of great arteries
  t. of great vessels
    (TGV)
**transseptal**
  t. angiocardiography
  t. catheter
  t. catheterization
  t. left heart
    catheterization
  t. puncture
**transthoracic pacing stylet**
**transvalvular flow**
**transvenous**
  t. device
  t. electrode
**transverse**
  t. incision
  t. section of heart
  t. tubule
**tranylcypromine**
**Trasicor**
**Trates**
**Traube's**
  T. bruit
  T. double tone
  T. sign
**trauma**
  blunt t.
**traumatic**
  t. aneurysm
  t. aortic aneurysm
  t. aortic disruption
  t. aortography
  t. asphyxia
  t. fistula

t. heart disease
t. rupture
t. tamponade
**trazodone**
t. hydrochloride
**Treacher Collins syndrome**
**treadmill**
exercise t.
t. test
**treatment**
Nauheim t.
Schott t.
**trefoil**
t. balloon
t. balloon catheter
t. catheter
**Trendelenburg position**
**Trendelenburg's**
T. operation
T. test
**Trental**
**trepidatio cordis**
**treponemal antibody**
*Treponema pallidum*
**trepopnea**
**treppe**
**Treppe's phenomenon**
**triad**
acute compression t.
Beck's t.
Fallot's t.
Hull's t.
Kartagener's t.
Osler's t.
**triadic junction**
**Trial**
Australian
Therapeutic T.
Coronary Primary
Prevention T. (CPPT)
**trial**
cardiac arrhythmia
suppression t. (CAST)

**triamterene**
**triangle**
Einthoven's t.
Koch's t.
**triatriatum**
cor t.
**triaxial reference system**
**triazolam**
**trichinosis**
**trichlormethiazide**
*Trichosporon*
**tricrotic**
**tricrotism**
**tricrotous**
**tricuspid**
t. area
t. atresia
t. incompetence
t. insufficiency
t. murmur
t. opening snap
t. position
t. regurgitation
t. restenosis
t. stenosis
t. valve
t. valve annulus
t. valve area
t. valve disease
t. valve doming
t. valve flow
t. valve prolapse
t. valve vegetation
t. valvuloplasty
**tricyclic antidepressant**
**Tridil**
**triethiodide**
gallamine t.
**trigeminal**
t. pulse
t. rhythm
**trigeminy**

**triggered**
    t. activity
    t. pacing
**triglyceride**
**triglyceride-rich lipoproteins
  (TRL)**
**trigone**
**triiodothyronine**
**trilazad mesylate**
**trileaflet**
**trilogy**
    t. of Fallot
**trimazosin**
**trimetaphan camsylate**
**trimethaphan**
**trimethoprim sulfate**
**trimipramine maleate**
**triphammer pulse**
**triphosphatase**
**triphosphate**
    adenosine t. (ATP)
**triple**
    t. balloon valvuloplasty
    t. rhythm
**triplets**
**tripolar w/Damato curve
  catheter**
**trisection**
    pulse t.
**tris(hydroxymethyl)aminomethane**
**trisomy**
    t. 13
    t. 18
    t. 21
**TRL**
    triglyceride-rich lipoproteins
**trochocardia**
**trochorizocardia**
**trophoblastic tumor**
**tropical endomyocardial
  fibrosis**
**tropomyosin**
**troponin**
    t. C

    t. I
    t. T
**trousers**
    military anti-shock t.
      (MAST)
    pneumatic t.
**Trousseau's syndrome**
**true**
    t. aortic aneurysm
    t. vs. false aneurysm
      aortography
**true-negative test result**
**true-positive test result**
**Truflex**
**trunci**
**truncoaortic sac**
**truncoconal area**
**truncus**, gen. and pl. **trunci**
    t. arteriosus
    persistent t. arteriosus
**Trunecek's symptom**
**trunk**
    bifurcation of
      pulmonary t.
    t. forward flexion
*Trypanosoma*
    *T. cruzi*
    *T. gambiense*
    *T. rhodesiense*
**trypanosomiasis**
**T sign**
**T system**
**TT**
    thrombin time
**Tubbs dilator**
**tube**
    bulboventricular t.
    Charnley drain t.
    endocardial t.
    Gore-Tex t.
    heart t.
    x-ray t.
**tuberculoid myocarditis**

**tuberculosis**
> renal t.

*tuberculosis*
> *Mycobacterium t.*

**tuberculous pericarditis**
**tuberoeruptive xanthoma**
**tuberous**
> t. sclerosis
> t. xanthoma

**tubocurarine chloride**
**tubular necrosis**
**tubule**
> distal convoluted t.
> proximal t.
> proximal convoluted t.
> transverse t.

**tug, tugging**
> tracheal t.

**tumor**
> carcinoid t.
> cardiac t.
> chromaffin cell t.
> t. embolism
> granular cell t.
> myxoma t.
> t. necrosis factor (TNF)
> papillary t.
> paraganglioma t.
> pericardiac t.
> phantom t.
> t. plop
> polycystic t.
> sarcomatous t.
> teratoma t.
> thyroid t.
> trophoblastic t.

**tumultus cordis**
**tunnel**
> percutaneous t.

**tunneler**
> Kelly-Wick vascular t.

**Tuohy-Bost**
> T.-B. adapter
> T.-B. introducer

**turbulence**
**turgor**
> coronary vascular t.

**Turner's syndrome**
**T vector**
**TVG**
> time-varied gain

**T wave**
**T-wave**
> inverted T-w.

**twiddler's syndrome**
**two-chamber view**
**two-dimensional**
> **echocardiography**

**two-step exercise test**
**Tylenol**
**type**
> t. A behavior
> t. B behavior
> cardioinhibitory t.
> t. 1 dextrocardia
> t. 2 dextrocardia
> t. 3 dextrocardia
> t. 4 dextrocardia
> t. I dip
> t. II dip

**typhoid fever**
**typhus**
> scrub t.

**typing**
> human lymphocyte
> antigen t.

**tyramine**
**tyrosine**

**ubiquitin**
**UD-CG 212**
**Uhl's**
    U. anomaly
    U. malformation
**ulcer**
    decubitus u.
    diabetic u.
    foot u.
    peptic u.
    stasis u.
    venous u.
**ulcerative**
    u. colitis
    u. endocarditis
**ulnar artery**
**ultimum moriens**
**ultracentrifugation**
**ultrafast computed tomography**
**Ultra-Select Nitinol PTCA**
  **guide wire**
**ultrasonographer**
**ultrasonography**
    Doppler u.
**ultrasonoscope**
**ultrasound**
    u. cardiography
    continuous-wave
     Doppler u.
    Doppler u.
    intravascular u. (IVUS)
**ultrastructure**
**umbilical**
    u. artery
    u. hernia
    u. tape
    u. vein
**umbrella**
    atrial septal defect u.
    Bard clamshell septal u.
    Bard PDA u.
    u. closure

    double u.
    patent ductus
     arteriosus u.
    PDA u.
    Rashkind double u.
**UMI transseptal Cath-Seal**
  **catheter introducer**
**underdrive pacing**
**undulating pulse**
**unicommissural**
**unidirectional block**
**unipolar**
    u. connector
    u. electrocardiogram
    u. leads
**Unistasis valve**
**unit**
    coronary care u. (CCU)
    digital fluoroscopic u.
    hybrid u.
    life change u.
    mobile coronary care u.
    peripheral resistance u.
     (PRU)
    R u.
    Wood u.
**univariate predictor**
**univentricular**
    u. atrioventricular
     connection
    u. heart
**universalis**
    adiposis u.
**universal pacemaker**
**Uniweave catheter**
**unstable**
    u. angina
    u. plaque
**upper**
    u. nodal extrasystole
    u. nodal rhythm
**upright exercise**

**upstairs-downstairs heart**
**upstroke**
    carotid u.
    diastolic u.
    u. velocity
**uptake**
    glucose u.
    myocardial oxygen u.
    oxygen u.
**urate**
**urea**
**Urecholine**
**uremia**
**uremic pericarditis**
**Uresil**
    U. embolectomy
      thrombectomy catheter
    U. radiopaque silicone
      band vessel loops

**urgency**
    hypertensive u.
**uric acid**
**urinary catheter**
**urine volume**
**urokinase**
**USCI**
    U. catheter
    U. Hyperflex guide wire
    U. introducer
**use dependence**
**U-shaped catheter loop**
**usurpation**
**Utah artificial heart**
**U wave**
**U wave alternans**

**V**$_{MAX}$
maximal velocity
**V-A**
ventriculoatrial
V-A conduction
V-A interval
**vaccine**
**vaccinia**
v. virus
**VAD**
ventricular assist device
**vagal**
v. attack
v. reaction
v. stimulation
**vagus**
v. nerve
v. pulse
**Valsalva**
V. maneuver
sinus of V.
V. test
**Valsalva's sinus**
**value**
index v.
predictive v.
reference v.
resting v.
**valve**
aortic v.
v. area
artificial v.
atrioventricular v.
ball v.
ball-cage v.
bicuspid aortic v.
bioprosthetic v.
Björk-Shiley v.
Braunwald-Cutter v.
caged-ball v.
cardiac v.
Carpentier-Edwards v.

cleft mitral v.
crisscross
atrioventricular v.
v. debris
diastolic fluttering
aortic v.
disc-cage v.
Duostat rotating
hemostatic v.
Duraflow heart v.
Ebstein's anomaly of
tricuspid v.
eustachian v.
flail mitral v.
floppy mitral v.
Hall-Kaster v.
heart v.
hemostasis v.
Kay-Shiley caged-disc v.
Lillehei-Kaster pivoting-
disc v.
mechanical v.
Medtronic-Hall v.
MH v.
mitral v.
Omnicarbon v.
Omniscience v.
v. orifice area
parachute v.
parachute mitral v.
porcine v.
porcine prosthetic v.
prosthetic v.
prosthetic aortic v.
prosthetic cardiac v.
pulmonary v.
pulmonic v.
v. replacement
v. rupture
semilunar v.
Smeloff heart v.
Starr-Edwards v.

**valve** *(continued)*
    St. Jude v.
    St. Jude Medical
      bileaflet v.
    straddling
      atrioventricular v.
    Surgitool prosthetic v.
    thebesian v.
    tilting-disk v.
    toroidal v.
    tricuspid v.
    Unistasis v.
**valvectomy**
**valvoplasty**
**valvotomy**
    aortic v.
    balloon v.
    balloon aortic v.
    balloon mitral v. (BMV)
    balloon pulmonary v.
    balloon tricuspid v.
    double-balloon v.
    v. knife
    mitral balloon v.
    mitral valve v.
    percutaneous balloon v.
    percutaneous mitral v.
    percutaneous mitral
      balloon v.
    repeat balloon mitral v.
    single balloon v.
**valvular**
    v. aortic stenosis
    v. calcification
    v. dysfunction
    v. endocarditis
    v. heart disease
    v. incompetence
    v. insufficiency
    v. regurgitation
    v. stenosis
    v. thrombus
**valvulitis**
    aortic v.

    mitral v.
    rheumatic v.
    syphilitic aortic v.
**valvuloplasty**
    aortic v.
    balloon v.
    balloon aortic v.
    balloon mitral v.
    balloon pulmonary v.
      (BPV)
    double-balloon v.
    intracoronary
      thrombolysis balloon v.
    mitral v.
    multiple balloon v.
    percutaneous balloon v.
    percutaneous balloon
      aortic v.
    percutaneous balloon
      pulmonic v.
    percutaneous mitral
      balloon v. (PMV)
    percutaneous
      transluminal balloon v.
    pulmonary v.
    pulmonic v.
    repeat balloon aortic v.
    repeat balloon
      pulmonary v.
    single balloon v.
    tricuspid v.
    triple balloon v.
**valvulotome**
**valvulotomy**
    aortic v.
**vanadium**
**vancomycin**
**Vaquez's disease**
**variability**
    baseline v. of fetal
      heart rate
**variable**
    v. coupling
    v. deceleration

**variance**
    ball v.
**variant**
    v. angina
    v. angina pectoris
**variation**
    beat-to-beat v. of fetal
        heart rate
**varicella**
**varices**
**varicose vein**
**varicosity**
    saphenous vein v.
**variola**
**Vario system**
**Varivas R denatured
  homologous vein graft**
**varix, pl. varices**
**Vascor**
**VascuClamp**
    V. minibulldog vessel
        clamp
    V. vascular clamp
**vascular**
    v. access catheter
    v. clamp
    v. clip
    v. graft prosthesis
    v. impedance
    v. incident
    v. injury
    v. murmur
    v. peripheral resistance
    v. redistribution
    v. resistance
    v. resistance index
    v. ring
    v. sclerosis
    v. sheath
    v. spasm
    v. stenosis
**vascularization**
**vasculature**
    pulmonary v.

**vasculitis**
    hypersensitivity v.
    leukocytoblastic v.
    necrotizing v.
    pulmonary v.
**vasculocardiac syndrome of
  hyperserotonemia**
**vasculopathy**
**vasoactive drug**
**vasoconstriction**
    pulmonary v.
**vasoconstrictor**
**vasodepression**
**vasodepressor syncope**
**vasodilation, vasodilatation**
    coronary v.
    reflex v.
**vasodilator**
    v. agent
    v. reserve
**Vasoglyn**
**vasomotion**
    coronary v.
**vasomotor**
    v. angina
    v. paralysis
**vasopressin**
    arginine v.
**vasopressor deficiency**
**vasoregulatory asthenia**
**vasospasm**
    coronary v.
**Vasotec**
**vasovagal**
    v. attack
    v. hypotension
    v. reaction
    v. syncope
    v. syndrome
**Vasoxyl**
**VATER**
    vertebral defects,
        imperforate anus,

**VATER** *(continued)*
  transesophageal fistula, and
  radial and renal dysplasia
    VATER association
    syndrome
    VATER complex
**VAT pacing**
**VCF**
  velocity of circumferential
  fiber shortening
**VCG**
  vectorcardiography
**VDD pacing**
**VDRL**
  Venereal Disease Research
  Laboratories
    VDRL test
**vector**
  v. cardiogram
  v. cardiography
  instantaneous v.
  v. loop
  manifest v.
  mean v.
  P v.
  QRS v.
  spatial v.
  T v.
**vectorcardiogram**
**vectorcardiography (VCG)**
  spatial v.
**vecuronium**
**vegetation**
  aortic valve v.
  endocardial v.
  prosthetic valve v.
  pulmonary valve v.
  tricuspid valve v.
  ventricular septal
    defect v.
**vegetative endocarditis**
**veiled puff**
**veiling glare**

**vein**
  allantoic v.
  anomalous pulmonary v.
  axillary v.
  azygos v.
  basilic v.
  brachial v.
  brachiocephalic v.
  cardiac v.
  cardinal v.
  cephalic v.
  coronary v.
  external jugular v.
  facial v.
  femoral v.
  v. graft
  v. graft cannula
  v. graft ring marker
  hemiazygos v.
  hepatic v.
  iliac v.
  internal jugular v.
  interventricular v.'s
  jugular v.
  left internal jugular v.
  Marshall's v.
  Marshall's oblique v.
  omphalomesenteric v.
  portal v.
  pulmonary v.
  renal v.
  saphenous v.
  subclavian v.
  thebesian v.
  umbilical v.
  varicose v.
  ventricular v.
  vitelline v.
**Velex woven Dacron vascular graft**
**velocardiofacial syndrome**
**velocity**
  aortic jet v.

# Got a Good Word for STEDMAN'S?

Help us keep STEDMAN'S products fresh and up-to-date with new words and new ideas!

Do we need to add or revise any items? Is there a better way to organize the content?

*Be specific!* How can we make this STEDMAN'S product the best medical word reference possible for you? Fill in the lines below with your thoughts and recommendations. Attach a separate sheet of paper if you need to— *you* are our most important contributor and we want to know what's on *your* mind. Thanks!

(PLEASE TYPE OR PRINT CAREFULLY)

Terms you believe are incorrect:

Appears as:                  Suggested revision:

_____

_____

_____

New terms you would like us to add:

_____

_____

Other comments:

_____

_____

_____

All done? Great, just mail this card in today. No postage necessary, and thanks again!

Name / Title:

Facility / Company:

Address:

City / State / Zip:

Day Telephone No. (          )

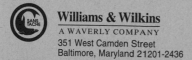

**Williams & Wilkins**
A WAVERLY COMPANY
351 West Camden Street
Baltimore, Maryland 21201-2436

*To order or to receive a catalog call toll free 1-800-527-5597.*

#079530–CARD

v. catheter technique
v. of circumferential
   fiber shortening (VCF)
ejection v.
flow v.
left ventricular outflow
   tract v.
maximal v. ($V_{MAX}$)
shortening v.
v. of shortening
upstroke v.
**vena**, pl. **venae**
   v. contracta
**vena cava**, pl. **venae cavae**
   v.c. cannula
   v.c. clip
   inferior v.c. (IVC)
   superior v.c. (SVC)
**vena caval**
   v. c. obstruction
   v. c. syndrome
**venacavogram**
**venae**
**venae cavae**
**venectasia**
**Venereal Disease Research
   Laboratories (VDRL)**
**venoconstriction**
**Venofit medical compression
   stockings**
**Venoflex medical compression
   stockings**
**venogram**
**venography**
**venom**
   arthropod v.
   bee v.
   black widow spider v.
   scorpion v.
   snake v.
   spider v.
**venopressor**
**venorespiratory reflex**
**venosity**

**venostasis**
**venosus**
   ductus v.
   sinus v.
**venous**
   v. access
   v. cannula
   v. collateral
   v. congestion
   v. cutdown
   v. embolism
   v. flow measurement
   v. heart
   v. hum
   v. hyperemia
   v. hypertension
   v. insufficiency
   v. mesenteric vascular
      occlusion
   v. murmur
   v. pressure
   v. pulse
   v. puncture
   v. return
   v. return curve
   v. sheath
   v. smooth muscle
   v. spasm
   v. thromboembolism
   v. thrombosis
   v. ulcer
**venovenous dye dilution curve**
**Ventak**
   V. AICD pacemaker
   V. defibrillator
**ventilation**
   assisted v.
   mechanical v.
   mouth-to-mouth v.
   v. scintigraphy
**ventilation-perfusion**
   v.-p. ratio
   v.-p. relation
   v.-p. scan

**ventilator**
  Infrasonics v.
  Puritan Bennett v.
  Siemens v.
**ventilatory threshold**
**ventricle**
  double-inlet v.
  double-outlet left v.
  double-outlet right v.
  left v. (LV)
  right v. (RV)
  single v.
  suicide v.
**ventricular**
  v. aberration
  v. afterload
  v. aneurysm
  v. angiography
  v. arrhythmia
  v. assist device (VAD)
  v. asynchronous
    pacemaker
  v. bigeminy
  v. biopsy
  v. bradycardia
  v. capture
  v. capture threshold
  v. complex
  v. conduction
  v. contour
  v. contractility
  v. demand pacemaker
  v. depolarization
    abnormality
  v. dilation
  v. distensibility
  v. ectopy
  v. end-diastolic volume
  v. end-systolic pressure-
    volume relation
  v. escape
  v. extrasystole
  v. fibrillation
  v. filling

  v. filling pressure
  v. flutter
  v. function
  v. function curve
  v. fusion beat
  v. gradient
  v. hypertrophy
  v. inflow anomaly
  v. inflow tract
    obstruction
  v. inhibited pulse
    generator
  v. interdependence
  v. inversion
  v. mapping
  v. milk spot
  v. myxoma
  v. outflow tract
    obstruction
  v. pacing
  v. perforation
  v. performance
  v. plateau
  v. power
  v. preload
  v. premature beat
    (VPB)
  v. premature contraction
  v. pressure
  v. pressure-volume loop
  v. pulse amplitude
  v. pulsewidth
  v. reentry
  v. refractory period
  v. relaxation
  v. rhythm
  v. sensing configuration
  v. sensitivity
  v. septal defect (VSD)
  v. septal defect murmur
  v. septal defect
    vegetation
  v. septal rupture
  v. septum

v. standstill
v. synchronous pulse generator
v. systole
v. tachyarrhythmia
v. tachycardia
v. thrombus
v. triggered pulse generator
v. vein
v. volume
v. wall motion
v. wall shortening
v. wall stress
v. wall thinning
v. wave (V wave)
ventricularization
ventriculoarterial
   v. concordance
   v. coupling
   v. discordance
ventriculoatrial (V-A)
   v. conduction
ventriculographic catheter
ventriculography
   biplane v.
   contrast v.
   left v.
   radionuclide v.
ventriculophasic
ventriculopuncture
ventriculoradial dysplasia
ventriculoscopy
ventriculotomy
   encircling endocardial v.
Ventritex Cadence implantable cardioverter-defibrillator
Venturi
   V. effect
   V. wave
venule
vera
   polycythemia v.
verapamil HCl

Verelan
Veri-Flex guide wire
vermicular pulse
verruca, pl. verrucae
verrucous endocarditis
Versed
vertebral artery bypass graft
vertebral defects, imperforate anus, transesophageal fistula, and radial and renal dysplasia (VATER)
vertebrobasilar occlusive disease
vertical heart
vertigo
   laryngeal v.
very low-density lipoprotein
vesicle
   intermediary v.
vessel
   capacitance v.
   v. clamp
   collateral v.
   v. dilator
   femoral v.
   ghost v.
   great v.
   v. occlusion system
   renal blood v.
   retinal v.
   splanchnic v.
   thoracic v.
   transposition of great v.'s (TGV)
VEST left ventricular function detector
Veterans Administration Cooperative Study
viability
   myocardial v.
vibration disease
vibrocardiogram
video
   v. camera

**video** *(continued)*
 v. imaging
 v. loop
 v. monitor
 v. system
**videodensitometry**
**videotape recorder**
**view**
 apical v.
 field of v.
 five-chamber v.
 four-chamber v.
 ice-pick v.
 laid-back v.
 long axial oblique v.
 long-axis v.
 parasternal v.
 sagittal v.
 short-axis v.
 sitting-up v.
 subcostal v.
 suprasternal v.
 two-chamber v.
**viewer**
 film v.
**vigilance response**
**vincristine sulfate**
**vindesine**
**Vineberg's procedure**
**viral**
 v. hepatitis
 v. myocarditis
 v. pericarditis
**virus**
 ECHO v.
  enteric cytopathogenic
   human orphan virus
 enteric cytopathogenic
  human orphan v.
  (ECHO virus)
 Epstein-Barr v.
 human
  immunodeficiency v.
  (HIV)

 respiratory syncytial v.
 vaccinia v.
**visceral**
 v. larva migrans
 v. pericardiectomy
**viscosimeter**
 Ostwald v.
**viscosity**
 blood v.
**vise**
 hemodynamic v.
**Visken**
**Vista pacemaker**
**visual acuity**
**visualization**
 fluoroscopic v.
**Vitagraft**
 V. arteriovenous shunt
 V. vascular graft
**vital capacity**
**vitamin B**
**vitamin B$_1$**
**vitamin B$_6$**
**vitamin B$_{12}$**
**vitamin C**
**vitamin D**
**vitamin K**
**vitamin K antagonist**
**Vitatron leads**
**vitelline vein**
**vitiligo**
 symmetric v.
**vitreous opacity**
**Vivactil**
**Vivalith II pulse generator**
**V lead**
**V. Mueller catheter**
**vocational rehabilitation**
**volt**
 electron v.
 kiloelectron v. (keV)
 megaelectron v. (MeV)
**voltage**
 v. criteria

v. equilibrium
transmembrane v.
**voltage-dependent calcium
channel**
**volume**
blood v.
cardiac v.
v. of distribution
$dP/dt_{MAX}$-end-diastolic v.
end-diastolic v. (EDV)
end-systolic v. (ESV)
intravascular v.
left ventricular v.
left ventricular end-
diastolic v.
left ventricular stroke v.
v. load hypertrophy
v. loading
mean corpuscular v.
(MCV)
v. overload
plasma v.
presystolic pressure
and v.
relative cardiac v.
v. stiffness
stroke v.
total blood v. (TBV)
urine v.

ventricular v.
ventricular end-
diastolic v.
**volume-challenge test**
**volume-time curve**
**vomiting**
**von Recklinghausen's disease**
**von Willebrand**
v. W. disease
v. W. factor
**voodoo death**
**VOO pacing**
**Voorhees bag**
**voussure**
**VPB**
ventricular premature beat
**VSD**
ventricular septal defect
**vulnerable**
v. period
v. period of heart
v. phase
**VVI pacing**
**VVIR pacing**
**VVT pacing**
**V wave**
ventricular wave
**V-waves**

waist
    w. of heart
**walk-through angina**
**wall**
    w. amplitude
    chest w.
    left ventricular w.
    w. motion
    w. motion analysis
    w. motion score
    w. motion study
    w. stress
    w. structure
    w. tension
    w. thickening
    w. thickness
**Wall stent**
**wandering**
    w. heart
    w. pacemaker
*Wangiella*
**warfarin**
    w. sodium
    w. therapy
**warm-up phenomenon**
**wash bath**
**wasp sting**
**wasting**
    potassium w.
    salt w.
**water**
    w. retention
    w. wheel murmur
**water-bottle heart**
**water-hammer pulse**
**watershed infarction**
**Waterston-Cooley procedure**
**Waterston shunt**
**Waterston's operation**
**Watson heart value holder**
**Watson's syndrome**

**wave**
    A w.
    *a*-w.
    arterial w.
    *c* w.
    cannon a w.
    cannon w.
    delta w.
    dicrotic w.
    electrocardiographic w.
    F w.
    f w.
    fibrillary w.'s
    flutter-fibrillation w.'s
    w. form
    h w.
    Osborne w.
    overflow w.
    P w.
    percussion w.
    postextrasystolic T w.
    pressure w.
    pulse w.
    Q w.
    R w.
    rapid filling w.
    recoil w.
    regurgitant w.
    retrograde P w.
    S w.
    T w.
    tidal w.
    U w.
    ventricular w. (V wave)
    Venturi w.
*a* **wave**
**waveform**
    pressure w.
**wavelength**
**weakness**
**Weber-Christian disease**
**Weber-Osler-Rendu syndrome**

Weber's experiment
Wedensky effect
wedge
    w. pressure
    w. pressure balloon
      catheter
wedged pulmonary angiography
Wegener's granulomatosis
weight
Weil's disease
Wenckebach
    W. atrioventricular block
    W. cycle
    W. period
Wenckebach's phenomenon
Werner's syndrome
Westermark sign
West's syndrome
wet beriberi
Wexler catheter
Wheatstone bridge
wheezing
whip
    catheter w.
White
    W. system for pediatric
      percutaneous
      catheterization
white
    w. blood cell count
    w. spot
    w. thrombus
Wholey
    W. Hi-torque modified
    J guide wire
    W. wire
whoop
    systolic w.
wide-complex tachycardia
wide QRS tachycardia
Wilkie's disease
William Harvey
    W. H. arterial blood
      filter

W. H. cardiotomy
    reservoir
Williams syndrome
Wilson
    W. block
    W. central terminal
Wilson-Cook papillotome
Wilson's disease
Windkessel effect
window
    aortic w.
    aorticopulmonary w.
    aortopulmonary w.
    cycle-length w.
    pericardial w.
    tachycardia w.
winged baseplate
Winiwarter-Buerger disease
winter bronchitis
wire
    ACS microglide w.
    AES Amplatz guide w.
    Amplex guide w.
    atherolytic reperfusion
     guide w.
    Becton-Dickinson
     guide w.
    Bentson exchange
     straight guide w.
    catheter guide w.
    central core w.
    control w.
    curved j-exchange w.
    delivery w.
    Elastorc catheter
     guide w.
    exchange guide w.
    floppy guide w.
    floppy tip guide w.
    guide w.
    w. guide
    guide w. loop
    guide w. perforation

Hancock temporary
  cardiac pacing w.
heparin-coated guide w.
high-torque w.
Hi-Per Flex w.
Hi-Per Flex exchange w.
Hi-Torque floppy
  exchange guide w.
Hi-Torque intermediate
  guide w.
w. holder
hydrophilic coated
  guide w.
w. insertion
J-exchange w.
J-guide w.
J Rosen guide w.
J-tip guide w.
Linx w.
Linx extension w.
Medi-Tech guide w.
Newton guide w.
PDT guide w.
Phantom w.
Phantom guide w.
Radifocus catheter
  guide w.
Reflex SuperSoft
  steerable guide w.
safety guide w.
silk guide w.
stainless steel w.
stainless steel guide w.
Teflon-coated guide w.
Terumo guide w.
Terumo "m" w.

tip-deflecting w.
Ultra-Select Nitinol
  PTCA guide w.
USCI Hyperflex
  guide w.
Veri-Flex guide w.
Wholey w.
Wholey Hi-torque
  modified J guide w.
**wiry pulse**
**Wolff-Parkinson-White (WPW)**
  W.-P.-W. bypass tract
  W.-P.-W. syndrome
**Wolvek sternal approximation**
  **fixation instrument**
**wooden-shoe heart**
**Wood unit**
**Woodworth's phenomenon**
**work**
  w. capacity
  w. rehabilitation
  w. status
  stroke w.
  w. threshold
**workers' compensation**
**wound**
  bullet w.
  entrance w.
  exit w.
  gunshot w.
  knife w.
  stab w.
**WPW**
  Wolff-Parkinson-White
**Wydora**
**Wytensin**

# X

xamoterol
xanthelasma
xanthogranuloma
xanthoma
    eruptive x.
    palmar x.
    x. striatum palmare
    x. tendinosum
    tendinous x.
    tuberoeruptive x.
    tuberous x.
x descent
Xe
    xenon
$^{133}$Xe
    xenon-133
$^{127}$Xe
    xenon-127
XeCl
    xenon chloride
      XeCl excimer laser
      XeCl laser
        xenon chloride laser

xenodiagnosis
xenograft
xenon (Xe)
    x. chloride (XeCl)
    x. chloride laser (XeCl
    laser)
    x. lung ventilation
    imaging
xenon-127 ($^{127}$Xe)
xenon-133 ($^{133}$Xe)
xipamide
XO syndrome
x-ray
    x.-r. beam filtration
    chest x.-r.
    x.-r. cine computed
    tomography
    x.-r. generator
    x.-r. system
    x.-r. tube
XXXX syndrome
XXXY syndrome
Xylocaine

# Y

YAG laser
Y-connector
    ACS angioplasty Y.-c.
y descent

yeast
yellow fever
*Yersinia*
YM 151

*Zuma guiding cath.*

**Z**

**Zaroxolyn**
**Z band**
**zero-order kinetics**
**Zestoretic**
**Zestril**
**Zimmer antiembolism**
  **stockings**
**zinc**
**Z line**
**Zocor**
**zofenopril**
**zone**
  Fraunhofer z.

  Fresnel z.
  H z.
  protective z.
  subendocardial z.
  transitional cell z.
**zoster**
  herpes z.
**Zucker**
  Z. catheter
  Z. multi-purpose bipolar
    catheter
**zygomycosis**

# Appendix 1
## Cardiac Catheterization

angled pigtail catheter
angulation
aortic pullback pressure
aspirated and flushed
atherosclerotic aortic disease
atherosclerotic narrowing
atrioventricular node (AVN)
AVN — atrioventricular node
Bruce protocol
CABG — coronary artery
  bypass graft
Cardizem
Cardizem CD
catheter
CHD — coronary heart
  disease
cineangiogram
circulation
circumflex (CX)
CK — creatine kinase
coronary artery bypass graft
  (CABG)
coronary heart disease (CHD)
creatine kinase (CK)
CX — circumflex
first obtuse marginal artery
  (OM-1)
flash-lamp excited pulsed dye
floppy guide wire
fluoroscopic visualization
fusiform aneurysm
global left ventricular ejection
  fraction
GUSTO protocol
Hartzler dilatation catheter
Hemashield
heparinized saline
iatrogenic atrial septal defect

Inoue balloon catheter
intraluminal
Judkins-Sones technique of
  cardiac catheterization
LAD — left axis deviation
LAO — left anterior oblique
LAO position
late reperfusion
left anterior oblique (LAO)
left axis deviation (LAD)
left dominant coronary
  circulation
left internal mammary artery
  (LIMA)
left ventricle (LV)
left ventricular end-diastolic
  pressure (LVEDP)
LIMA — left internal
  mammary artery
LV — left ventricle
LVEDP — left ventricular
  end-diastolic pressure
millijoule (mJ)
mitral valve area (MVA)
mitral valve gradient (MVG)
mJ — millijoule
modified Bruce protocol
MVA — mitral valve area
MVG — mitral valve
  gradient
needle
New York Heart Association
  (NYHA)
New York Heart Association
  classification
no-reflow phenomenon
NYHA — New York Heart
  Association

occlusion
OM-1 — first obtuse
  marginal artery
OM-2 — second obtuse
  marginal artery
opacify
ostium
peak systolic aortic pressure
  (PSAP)
peak systolic gradient (PSG)
percutaneous mitral balloon
  valvotomy
percutaneous mitral balloon
  valvuloplasty (PMV)
peripheral atherosclerotic
  disease
PMV — percutaneous mitral
  balloon valvuloplasty
port
position
pressure
PSAP — peak systolic aortic
  pressure
PSG — peak systolic
  gradient
PSG pressure

pullback pressure
Quinidex
ramus intermedius artery
RAO — right anterior
  oblique
RAO angulation
RAO position
right anterior oblique (RAO)
saline
scattergram
second obtuse marginal artery
  (OM-2)
sheath
side port
single-photon emission
sinus node (SN)
SN — sinus node
stenosis
technetium-99m imaging
thallium-201 stress test
thrombolytic agent
USCI catheter
venous sheath
visualization
wire

# Appendix 2
## Percutaneous Transluminal Coronary Angioplasty (PTCA)

angioplasty
arterial sheath
ASC Alpha balloon
ASC RX perfusion balloon
  catheter
atheroblation laser
atrioventricular node (AVN)
AVN — atrioventricular node
balloon
balloon-centered argon laser
balloon pump
Baxter Intrepid balloon
Bruce protocol
CABG — coronary artery
  bypass graft
Cardizem
Cardizem CD
catheter
CHD — coronary heart
  disease
circumflex (CX)
CK — creatine kinase
coronary artery bypass graft
  (CABG)
coronary heart disease (CHD)
creatine kinase (CK)
CX — circumflex
dye
ECLA — excimer laser
  coronary angioplasty
Eppendorf catheter
excimer laser coronary
  angioplasty (ECLA)
first obtuse marginal artery
  (OM-1)
flash-lamp excited pulsed dye
floppy

fluorescence-guided "smart"
  laser
fraction
French JR4 Schneider
  catheter
French SAL catheter
French sheath
fusiform aneurysm
global left ventricular ejection
  fraction
Goodale-Lubin catheter
guider
guide wire
guiding catheter
hadow balloon
Hartzler dilatation catheter
helium-cadmium diagnostic
  laser
Hemashield
high-flow catheter
Hi-Per Flex wire
Hi-Torque floppy with Propel
holmium laser
hot-tip laser probe
iatrogenic atrial septal defect
Inoue balloon catheter
intra-aortic balloon
intraluminal
intravascular ultrasound
  (IVUS)
introducer
IVUS — intravascular
  ultrasound
J-guide wire
JR4 catheter
JR5 catheter

**Judkins-Sones technique of cardiac catheterization**
**Kay balloon**
**LAD** — left axis deviation
**laser**
**late reperfusion**
**left axis deviation (LAD)**
**left internal mammary artery (LIMA)**
**left ventricle (LV)**
**left ventricular end-diastolic pressure (LVEDP)**
**lens**
**LIMA** — left internal mammary artery
**Linx extension wire**
**LV** — left ventricle
**LVEDP** — left ventricular end-diastolic pressure
**manifold**
**MB fraction**
**Medi-Tech balloon catheter**
**millijoule (mJ)**
**mitral valve area (MVA)**
**mitral valve gradient (MVG)**
**mJ** — millijoule
**modified Bruce protocol**
**MVA** — mitral valve area
**MVG** — mitral valve gradient
**Mylar catheter**
**Nd:YAG laser** — neodymium:yttrium-aluminum-garnet laser
**neodymium:yttrium-aluminum-garnet laser (Nd:YAG laser)**
**Nestor-3**
**Nestor guiding catheter**
**New York Heart Association (NYHA)**
**New York Heart Association classification**
**NL3 guider**
**NoProfile balloon**

**no-reflow phenomenon**
**NYHA** — New York Heart Association
**occlusion**
**Olbert balloon**
**OM-1** — first obtuse marginal artery
**OM-2** — second obtuse marginal artery
**opacify**
**ostium**
**peak systolic aortic pressure (PSAP)**
**peak systolic gradient (PSG)**
**percutaneous mitral balloon valvotomy**
**percutaneous mitral balloon valvuloplasty (PMV)**
**Phantom guide wire**
**Phantom wire**
**PMV** — percutaneous mitral balloon valvuloplasty
**probe**
**Propel**
**PSAP** — peak systolic aortic pressure
**PSG** — peak systolic gradient
**PSG pressure**
**pullback pressure**
**pump**
**Quinidex**
**radiocontrast dye**
**ramus intermedius artery**
**rotational ablation laser**
**sapphire lens**
**scattergram**
**second obtuse marginal artery (OM-2)**
**sheath**
**silk guide wire**
**single-photon emission**
**sinus node (SN)**
**Skinny balloon catheter**

# Percutaneous Transluminal Coronary Angioplasty (PTCA)

**Slinky balloon**
**SN** — sinus node
**spectroscopy-directed laser**
**spirometer**
**stenosis**
**TEC** — transluminal extraction-endarterectomy catheter
**technetium-99m imaging**
**thallium-201 stress test**

**thrombolytic agent**
**tip-deflecting wire**
**Tissot spirometer**
**transluminal extraction-endarterectomy catheter (TEC)**
**ultrasound**
**USCI introducer**
**wire**

# Appendix 3
## Carotid Endarterectomy

angiography
ansa cervicalis
arteriotomy
backbleeding
bifurcation
blunt eversion carotid
  endarterectomy
carotid artery
carotid Doppler
carotid endarterectomy
carotid sheath
cerebral perfusion
common carotid artery
endarterectomy
external jugular vein
facial vein
heparinization
hypoglossal nerve
internal carotid artery
internal jugular vein
intima

intimal flap
jugular vein
lumina
luminal narrowing
Model 40-400 Pruitt-Inahara
  shunt
plaque
platysma
Pruitt-Inahara shunt
reversible ischemic neurologic
  debility (RIND)
RIND — reversible ischemic
  neurologic debility
Rumel tourniquet
stenosis
sternocleidomastoid
superior carotid artery
superior thyroid artery
umbilical tape
vertigo